Diabetes: Emergency and Hospital Management

Simon R Page

Consultant Physician, Department of Diabetes,
Endocrinology and Nutrition,
Queen's Medical Centre, Nottingham

George M Hall

Professor of Anaesthesia, St George's Hospital
Medical School, London

© BMJ Books 1999
BMJ Books is an imprint of the BMJ Publishing Group

First published in 1999
by BMJ Books, BMA House, Tavistock Square,
London WC1H 9JR

British Library Cataloguing in Publication Data

A catalogue record for this book is available from the
British Library

ISBN 0-7279-1229-1

Typeset, printed and bound in Great Britain by
Latimer Trend & Company Ltd, Plymouth

Diabetes: Emergency and Hospital Management

Contents

Preface

Patients with diabetes occupy one in ten hospital beds in developed countries and consume a disproportionately large slice of health care expenditure. Commonly, admissions are a direct result of diabetes or its complications but even when the admission is not directly related to diabetes, hospital staff must decide how the condition should be managed and "troubleshoot" problems as they arise on hospital wards.

The main intention in writing this book was to provide a guide to the management of diabetes in the hospital setting mainly aimed at the non-specialist doctor. In most hospitals it is the junior doctors who are the "front line" troops involved in the diagnosis and management of emergency admissions and it is junior doctors who, with anaesthetic colleagues, manage patients with diabetes who require emergency or elective surgery.

The initial chapters describe essential background information about diabetes and its treatment, mainly focusing on blood glucose control. Guidelines for managing diabetes in hospital wards are provided in Chapter 2 to help the junior doctor who is faced with the all too common request from a ward nurse to review a patient with diabetes who has been found to have a blood glucose of 20 mmol/litre.

The diagnosis and management of acute metabolic problems including ketoacidosis, hyperosmolar non-ketotic coma and hypoglycaemia are described in the following two chapters. Chapter 5 describes the management of the diabetic patient before, during and after emergency, elective and day-case surgery and we have included guidelines on diabetes management during common investigations since we have found that such practical advice is difficult to find in standard textbooks of diabetes.

The remaining chapters aim to cover the common and less common systems based complications of diabetes, which usually require hospital admission or assessment. These include discussion of the management of myocardial infarction in diabetic patients, the diabetic foot, eye and renal complications and infections. In addition to management guidelines each of these chapters provide a theoretical and where possible evidence-based discussion of the complications of diabetes, together with illustrative case studies which highlight management issues in a clinically relevant way.

We hope this book can form a basis for drawing up local management guidelines to help junior hospital doctors to diagnose, investigate and treat diabetic patients during a hospital admission.

We are grateful to Professor Robert Tattersall for his extremely helpful comments on the manuscript and for providing some of the ideas for case studies. We also wish to thank our publishers, and, in particular Mary Banks, Senior Commissioning Editor for her patience as several deadlines for receipt of the manuscript passed by. I (SRP) would also wish to acknowledge the forbearance of my family as my attention became increasingly focused on my computer screen over many evenings and weekends.

1 Diagnosis, classification, and pathophysiology of diabetes

To manage a condition rationally, you must understand its aetiology, pathophysiology, and treatment. This chapter summarises key features in the presentation, diagnosis, and management of diabetes and sets the scene for the rest of the book.

Definition

Diabetes mellitus is a diverse disorder: its main presentation is chronic hyperglycaemia, caused by *either* insulin deficiency *or* resistance to the effects of insulin in peripheral tissues *or a combination of these*. The diagnostic criteria of the World Health Organisation (1985) are based on plasma (or whole blood) glucose measurement:[1]

- A single random plasma glucose of $\geqslant 11.1$ mmol/litre, or a fasting value of $\geqslant 7.8$ mmol/litre in a symptomatic but "well" patient is sufficient to confirm the diagnosis.
- A fasting or random plasma glucose <5.5 mmol/litre excludes the diagnosis.
- A random glucose between 5.5 and 11.0 mmol/litre is inconclusive. A fasting plasma glucose should be done and interpreted as above. With a fasting glucose between 5.5 and 7.7 mmol/litre, a 75 g oral glucose tolerance test (OGTT) may be needed. The criteria for interpretation are shown in Table 1.1.

1

Table 1.1 Diagnostic criteria for diabetes and impaired glucose tolerance following a 75 g oral glucose tolerance test

Sample	Diabetes		Impaired glucose tolerance	
	Fasting	2-hour	Fasting	2-hour
	(mmol/litre)		(mmol/litre)	
Plasma	⩾7.8	⩾11.1	<7.8	7.8–11.0
Whole blood	⩾6.7	⩾10.0	<6.7	6.7–9.9

Whilst acknowledging the above criteria, the American Diabetes Association has recently recommended modifications based on measurement of the plasma glucose after an 8-hour fast mainly for epidemiological and screening purposes.[2] Under these recommendations, a fasting plasma glucose of ⩾7.0 mmol/litre (126 mg/dl) enables a provisional diagnosis of diabetes to be made, a value of <6.0 mmol/litre (110 mg/dl) is defined as a normal fasting glucose, and a value of ⩾6.0 mmol/litre and <7.0 mmol/litre (⩾110 and <126 mg/dl respectively) is provided with a new classification of impaired fasting glucose. These new diagnostic criteria are currently under review by the WHO, and have not (yet) been accepted.

Classification

The WHO classification of diabetes defines two major types according to whether insulin therapy is essential for survival (type 1 diabetes; insulin-dependent diabetes; IDDM) or not (type 2 diabetes; non-insulin-dependent diabetes; NIDDM):[1]

Clinical classes

- *Diabetes mellitus*
  - Type 1 (insulin-dependent diabetes, IDDM)
  - Type 2 (non-insulin-dependent diabetes, NIDDM)
    - obese
    - non-obese
  - Diabetes related to other conditions (see text)
  - Gestational diabetes mellitus (GDM)
  - Malnutrition-related diabetes

- *Impaired glucose tolerance (IGT)*
  - obese
  - non-obese
- Related to other conditions

Statistical risk classes

- *Previous abnormality of glucose tolerance*
- *Potential abnormality of glucose tolerance*

Classifying a complex and heterogeneous disorder in this rather simplistic way inevitably has drawbacks and may lead to incorrect clinical assumptions. For example, about one in five patients with type 2 diabetes needs insulin to control hyperglycaemia. This does not mean that they have become "dependent" since withdrawal of insulin will lead to hyperglycaemia but not ketoacidosis, the cardinal sign of type 1 diabetes. They should be classified as insulin-treated type 2 rather than type 1 diabetes, a distinction which can be important when you are planning management during surgery or intercurrent illness. The interval between diagnosis of diabetes and starting insulin is a good guide; in insulin-treated type 2 diabetes this is usually longer than a year.

Some patients with type 2 diabetes may become temporarily "insulin-dependent" during severe intercurrent illness as illustrated in the following case report.

Case Study 1

A 55-year-old woman with long-standing type 2 diabetes, normally well controlled on gliclazide and metformin, was admitted with a 2-day history of vomiting, diarrhoea, and dehydration. She had become more unwell on the day of admission with shortness of breath and a reduced level of consciousness.

On arrival she was drowsy with acidotic breathing and a fever of 38°C. There was an area of cellulitis in her groin. Initial investigations confirmed a glucose of 31.8 mmol/litre, a low venous bicarbonate of 11 mmol/litre (normal range 24–30 mmol/litre) and heavy ketonuria. The arterial pH was 7.16.

She was treated with intravenous fluids, potassium, and insulin, together with broad spectrum antibiotics. Over the next 2 days her insulin requirements averaged 120 units/day. The area of cellulitis worsened despite treatment and she required extensive surgical debridement of infected necrotic subcutaneous tissue. Post-operatively her temperature settled and her insulin requirements

3

fell to 30 units/day with good blood glucose control. She was maintained on subcutaneous insulin until the surgical site began to heal. She then successfully restarted diet and tablets.

This case illustrates that, whilst insulin may be needed during the illness to prevent ketogenesis and hyperglycaemia, on recovery patients are usually able to resume their previous treatment for type 2 diabetes.

The WHO classification also recognises less common causes of diabetes which can be grouped under the broad headings of *pancreatic disease, endocrine disease, genetic disorders* and *drug-related*. In the following sections the pathophysiology of each type of diabetes will be described in more detail.

Pathophysiology

Type 1 diabetes

Type 1 diabetes is a chronic autoimmune disease in which the insulin-producing β-cells of the islets of Langerhans are progressively destroyed. About 70% of cases present under 30 years of age with a peak in adolescence of about 20 per 100 000 cases per year in the UK. It is important to remember that one-third present over 30 years of age; in fact type 1 diabetes is just as likely to present in an 80-year-old as a 40-year-old.[3]

What causes type 1 diabetes?

Genetic, environmental and immunological factors are involved. Evidence for a genetic predisposition has come from studies in twins[4] and in associations with class II histocompatibility (HLA) antigens.[5]

Environmental factors have been implicated with:

- viral infection (Cocksackie B4, intrauterine rubella infection);
- toxins (nitroso-compounds);
- constituents of the diet (cow's milk exposure in infancy)

but the environmental trigger(s) remains unknown.

The hallmark of type 1 diabetes is a chronic immune cell infiltrate in the islets of Langerhans causing the selective destruction of β-cells.[6] Both humoral and cellular immunity are involved. Humoral immunity is characterised by a polyclonal IgG antibody

4

response against several autoantigens. Islet cell antibodies can be detected up to 10 years before clinical presentation.

Symptomatic disease

By the time typical symptoms develop, over 90% of β-cells have been destroyed causing marked insulin deficiency, the hallmark of type 1 diabetes. To make matters worse, hyperglycaemia prevents the remaining β-cells from working normally, an effect termed *glucose toxicity*. The combined effects of insulin deficiency and glucose toxicity cause the relatively dramatic presentation of type 1 diabetes.

Glucose toxicity is reversible in the short term. Control of hyperglycaemia with insulin helps the remaining β-cells to work better for a few months after diagnosis. This is the basis of the *honeymoon period* when insulin doses are small (see Chapter 2). Unfortunately, the autoimmune process continues until the β-cells have been destroyed and most patients have to increase their insulin doses about a year after diagnosis.

The newly diagnosed patient with type 1 diabetes

There is no easily available diagnostic test for type 1 diabetes and clinical features are crucial. The most helpful signs are:

- *moderate or heavy ketonuria* resulting from excessive fat metabolism and, in the presence of hyperglycaemia, is sufficient to confirm type 1 diabetes;
- *recent onset of severe symptoms* strongly suggestive with a patient typically taking jugs of water to bed and suffering nocturia several times each night;
- *marked weight loss over a few weeks*, irrespective of the patient's initial weight;
- *a history of type 1 diabetes in a first-degree relative*, or a personal history of other organ-specific autoimmune disease.

Two other points should be mentioned. First, diabetes developing in middle or old age *does not* automatically mean treatment with diet and tablets. One-third of patients with type 1 present over the age of 30, but the notion that middle or old age equates with tablets can lead to illogical clinical practice as illustrated in the following case:

Case Study 2

An 84-year-old woman was admitted to a general medical ward with nausea and vomiting. She had a blood glucose of 32.7 mmol/litre, a venous bicarbonate of 8 mmol/litre and +++urinary ketones. She was correctly treated with intravenous fluids and insulin, but once she was better she was put on a diet and oral hypoglycaemic tablets, and discharged. At follow-up 6 weeks later she continued to have symptoms, her urine tests remained positive, and she had lost 5 kg in weight. The dose of tablets was increased and she was referred to the diabetes team. At her next review her weight had fallen by a further 4 kg, and her urine showed heavy ketonuria. She was restarted on insulin the same day and within a few weeks had regained her weight and was in good health.

It has recently become clear that some patients may present with what seems like type 2 diabetes but have immunological features more typical of type 1 diabetes. Such patients probably have less aggressive immunological destruction of their β-cells, and this explains both the slow symptomatic onset and the fact that they can often be managed with diet and tablets for months or years before insulin treatment becomes inevitable. They are classified as LADA (not the Russian car, but Latent Autoimmune Diabetes of Adults).

Secondly, the height of the blood sugar is *unhelpful* in deciding the need for insulin. Although partly determined by insulin lack, blood glucose is also influenced by food intake and renal losses. Some patients who quench their thirst with glucose-containing drinks may have blood glucose levels >30 mmol/litre which respond rapidly to diet, whereas a patient with ketonuria may become acidotic within a few days with blood sugars remaining in the low teens.

Is insulin therapy needed immediately?

If a diagnosis of type 1 diabetes is suspected on clinical grounds, the answer is yes, irrespective of the patient's age. For patients who are not acutely unwell, working through the algorithm (Figure 1.1) will provide a logical approach to deciding the need for insulin. If in doubt, it is wise to start insulin, as it can always be stopped at a later date.

Previously undiagnosed type 1 diabetes may present with ketoacidosis, although this is becoming much less common in

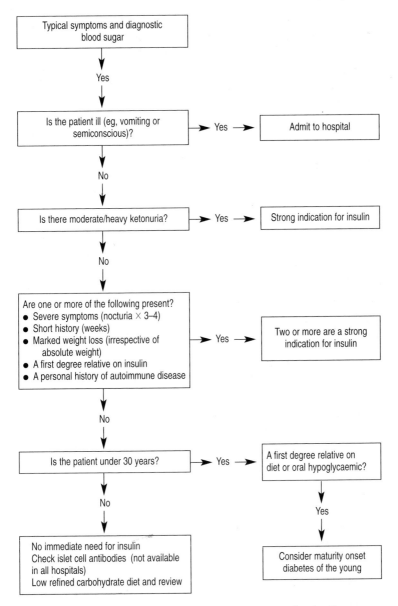

Figure 1.1   Algorithm for deciding whether a patient needs immediate insulin treatment.

developed countries because of the earlier recognition of the symptoms of diabetes. The management of ketoacidosis is described in Chapter 3.

In most cases the decision to start insulin is relatively straightforward, but occasionally, perhaps as a result of a routine urine test or medical insurance examination, diabetes is diagnosed in a patient under 30 years old who has few, if any, symptoms. There is no immediate need for insulin in such cases, but there are several reasons why early insulin treatment may be advisable:

- 95% will need insulin within 1 year;
- non-specific symptoms, such as fatigue, are only effectively treated with insulin;
- early insulin treatment may preserve β-cell function.

If the decision not to start insulin therapy is taken, it is vital that patients are shown how to test their urine for ketones, and provided with contact telephone numbers in the event of worsening symptoms or the development of ketonuria.

Type 2 diabetes

Type 2 diabetes accounts for 90% of cases of diabetes and affects 3% of the UK population. It is more common with increasing age, obesity, and in certain ethnic groups, affecting one in three Asians over 65 years of age, compared with one in 10 Caucasians. In Asians and Afro-Caribbeans, it presents, on average, 10 years earlier than in Caucasians.

What causes type 2 diabetes?

This is not completely understood, but both genetic and environmental factors are involved. Studies in twins, families, and racial groups provide evidence for genetic influences. In many cases it is probably inherited as a "polygenic" trait involving several different, as yet unidentified genes.

Several common environmental factors can contribute to the risk of developing type 2 diabetes (Table 1.2).

The relationship between genetic and environmental factors is complex. For example, obesity, a major risk factor, is partly genetically and partly environmentally determined. The situation is even more complex because genetic factors also influence the

Table 1.2   Common environmental factors contributing to the risk of developing type 2 diabetes

Factor	Comments
Age	Increases with age in all populations
Obesity	Two-thirds of patients are overweight
	Both genetic and environmental factors influence the development of obesity
	Risk is higher with central (android) obesity which is associated with greater insulin resistance than gynaecoid obesity
Inactivity	Causes increased insulin resistance
Birthweight	Small "undernourished" babies are at greatest risk in later life, possibly from reduced β-cell reserve resulting from malnutrition in the uterus during β-cell maturation.

distribution of excess fat. Weight gain around the abdomen (android), with a high waist–hip ratio, is associated with a greater risk than that around the hips (gynaecoid).

The pathophysiology of type 2 diabetes

Type 2 diabetes is a slowly progressive disease which results from a combination of insulin-insensitivity of target tissues, especially skeletal muscle, termed *insulin resistance*, and *relative insulin deficiency*.[7] The likely interaction between these factors is described below.

It is now accepted that insulin resistance predates the development of type 2 diabetes by many years, but it is not by itself sufficient to cause it. Up to 25% of the population have insulin resistance of a similar degree to people with type 2 diabetes and most respond by increasing insulin secretion to maintain normal blood glucose concentrations. However, some individuals cannot sustain hyperinsulinaemia and, with the progressive failure of the β-cell, blood sugar levels rise. Insulin deficiency results in increased glucose output from the liver, an important determinant of fasting glucose concentrations, and reduced peripheral uptake of glucose into skeletal muscle. Both are important factors in the development of hyperglycaemia. The relationship between insulin resistance and progressive hyperglycaemia is shown in Figure 1.2.

There is a marked difference in the sensitivity of different tissues to insulin, with inhibition of lipolysis occurring at very low insulin levels, whilst several-fold higher concentrations are needed to switch off hepatic gluconeogenesis. This is of clinical relevance because insulin deficiency is not generally as severe in type 2 diabetes as in type 1, and there is usually enough insulin to prevent ketogenesis, but not progressive hyperglycaemia.

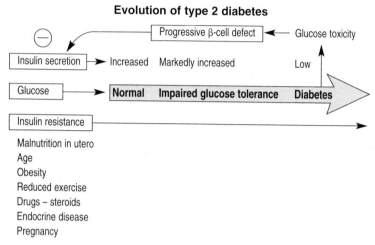

Figure 1.2   *Evolution of type 2 diabetes.*

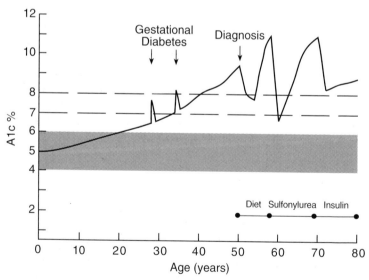

Figure 1.3   *Gradual development of hyperglycaemia in type 2 diabetes (with permission from Riddle[8]).*

It is also important to realise that type 2 diabetes may have a "preclinical" phase of five or more years (Figure 1.3) during which patients are exposed to an abnormal metabolic environment. This may explain why 50% of patients have both microvascular and/or macrovascular complications at diagnosis.

Unfortunately, insulin resistance or deficiency is impossible to measure in clinical practice, but in general terms insulin deficiency is likely to be the major factor in patients who are of normal weight or thin, whereas insulin resistance becomes much more important with increasing obesity. Although these are broad generalisations, they can be helpful in guiding clinical management. For example:

- Insulin doses during surgery or intercurrent illness are likely to be higher in overweight patients in order to overcome insulin resistance.
- Drugs, particularly glucocorticoids, increase insulin resistance and may precipitate or exacerbate diabetes.
- Overweight patients are also less likely to develop ketoacidosis, in the face of an intercurrent illness, than normal weight patients who are generally more insulin deficient.

The newly diagnosed patient with type 2 diabetes

Only 50% of patients present with typical hyperglycaemic symptoms. In some patients the diagnosis is made as a result of insurance checks or health checks. It can commonly be picked up during a hospital visit, for example during a preoperative assessment for elective surgery or during an emergency admission. Consider the following case study where the finding of previously unsuspected diabetes poses questions about diagnosis and management, and how the diagnosis will affect the planned operation.

Case Study 3

A 58-year-old overweight woman is seen during a surgical pre-admission assessment and is noted to have a blood glucose of 15.4 mmol/litre on routine testing. On questioning, she has been tired for several months but had put the symptoms down to stress. She had also had two episodes of vaginal thrush. Her mother had "late onset diabetes". She was due to be admitted for an elective laparoscopic cholecystectomy two weeks later, following two episodes of acute biliary colic over the last six months.

11

Box 1.1 Secondary causes of diabetes

● **Pancreatic disease**

Pancreatitis
Glucose intolerance in 50% with acute pancreatitis but only 2% need insulin after a single episode. Chronic pancreatitis complicated by diabetes in 45% of cases. Insulin eventually needed in 30%.

Cancer of pancreas
20% have IGT (impaired glucose tolerance) or diabetes. Useful clues include abdominal pain or continued weight loss despite good diabetic control.

Pancreatectomy
If total, causes insulin-dependent diabetes. Lack of glucagon increases sensitivity to insulin and risk of hypoglycaemia.

Cystic fibrosis
Autosomal recessive; prevalence 1 per 5000. Diabetes in 25% from pancreatic damage.

Haemochromatosis
Autosomal recessive. Increased iron absorption and deposition. Male predominance of 10:1. Abnormal liver function tests and hepatomegaly are typical but may be mistaken for a "fatty" liver in type 2 diabetes. Diabetes in 25% usually occurs in the fourth or fifth decade. Slate grey skin pigmentation from increased melanin. Diagnosis by liver biopsy. Serum transferrin saturation or ferritin are useful screening tests. Regular venesection does not cure diabetes, which usually requires insulin.

● **Endocrine disease**

Cushing's syndrome
Diabetes is present in 30%. Usually managed with diet and tablets. Effective treatment of Cushing's syndrome cures diabetes.

Acromegaly
Increased growth hormone, usually from a pituitary adenoma. Diabetes in 30%, usually diet and tablet controlled. Insulin occasionally needed.

continued

Box 1.1 *continued*

- **Endocrine disease**
  - *Hyperthyroidism*   Mild impairment of glucose tolerance, not usually of clinical significance. Rarely, thyroid storm can be associated with diabetic ketoacidosis in a patient with no past history of diabetes.
  - *Conn's syndrome*   Either an adrenal adenoma or bilateral adrenal hyperplasia. Hypertension and hypokalaemia are clinical manifestations. Since hypokalaemia impairs insulin release, up to 50% have abnormal glucose tolerance.
  - *Phaeochromocytoma*   Catecholamine-secreting tumour usually of the adrenal medulla. IGT in 75% because catecholamines increase hepatic glycogen breakdown and inhibit insulin release.
  - *Glucagonoma*   Slow-growing pancreatic tumour. Often metastasised to the liver at presentation. Increased glucagon secretion affects hepatic glucose metabolism causing diabetes.

- **Secondary causes of diabetes**
  - *Beta-blockers*   Impair insulin release. May cause impaired glucose tolerance or type 2 diabetes.
  - *Thiazide diuretics*   Hypokalaemia impairs insulin release. May cause impaired glucose tolerance or type 2 diabetes. Combination of beta-blockers and thiazide increase the risk by 10-fold.
  - *Diazoxide*   Inhibits insulin secretion. Occasionally used in the treatment of insulinoma.
  - *β_2-agonists*   Increase hepatic glucose output. Clinically important only if used in high doses intravenously.
  - *Glucocorticoids*   Increase hepatic glucose production and worsen insulin resistance. Dose-related effect. With high doses, insulin may be needed for control.

What effect will the diagnosis of diabetes have on elective surgery?

The diagnosis of diabetes prior to an operation requires reassessment of the management priorities: it is sensible to ensure that diabetes is as well controlled as possible before elective surgery is undertaken. The history and examination will indicate whether other problems, for example undiagnosed retinopathy, demand more urgent clinical attention and, where relevant, appropriate referral should be made. In the case of uncomplicated newly-diagnosed diabetes, a treatment plan should be started, including patient information, dietary advice, and instruction in urine or blood testing. This will probably involve local services for people with diabetes. Elective surgery should be reorganised once the diabetes is under control either with diet, tablets, or insulin as necessary. Treatment of diabetes is discussed in Chapter 2.

Secondary causes of diabetes

Secondary causes of diabetes, although uncommon, should be kept in mind when you are assessing new patients. They can be classified into pancreatic, endocrine, and drug-related (Box 1.1).

A number of genetic syndromes are associated with diabetes. Single gene mutations have recently been described in Maturity Onset Diabetes of the Young (MODY), a familial form of diabetes first described by Tattersall in 1974.[9] MODY usually presents in patients <25 years who do not have autoimmune markers of type 1 diabetes and who do not need insulin within five years of

---

Box 1.2 Genetic disorders associated with diabetes

• DIDMOAD	Diabetes insipidus, diabetes mellitus, optic atrophy and deafness. Diabetes mellitus develops in childhood and is ketosis prone.
• Myotonic dystrophy	About 10% have type 2 diabetes.
• Friedreich's ataxia	About 10% develop type 2 diabetes.
• Lipoatrophy	Can be partial or complete. Associated with markedly raised triglycerides and interstitial nephritis.

Box 1.3 Investigations needed in newly diagnosed people with diabetes

● Essential

● *Glucose*	Random or fasting to confirm the diagnosis according to current WHO criteria.
● *HBA1c*	As a baseline against which to judge response to treatment.
● *Creatinine*	To establish a baseline for renal function.
● *Electrolytes*	Hypokalaemia unexplained by diuretic treatment should raise the possibility of Cushing's or Conn's syndrome.
● *Urinalysis*	For glucose, protein, microalbumin and ketones.
● *ECG*	Baseline assessment.
● *Fasting lipids*	Type 2 diabetes is associated with abnormal lipid profiles. Fasting lipids should be measured once hyperglycaemia has been "stabilised". Patients often have raised LDL cholesterol and triglycerides, and low HDL-cholesterol concentrations.

● If clinically indicated

● *TFTs*	Worth checking in newly diagnosed patients with type 1 diabetes because of autoimmune associations. Only if clinically indicated in type 2 diabetes.
● *LFTs*	Up to 40% of newly diagnosed patients with type 2 diabetes have at least one abnormal test, which is usually due to fatty change. Worth checking if underlying alcohol-related problems or haemochromatosis suspected.
● *Ferritin*	If haemochromatosis is suspected clinically by hepatomegaly, hypogonadism, or skin pigmentation. Routine screening not justified.
● *Pancreatic imaging*	If there is a clinical suspicion of chronic pancreatitis or pancreatic carcinoma.
● *Overnight dexamethasone suppression test*	If clinical features of Cushing's syndrome present. Give 1 mg oral dexamethasone at 22.00 h; check plasma cortisol at 09.00 h next morning. A normal result would be a cortisol of <50 nmol/litre. Inadequate suppression should prompt further investigation (**seek advice**).
● *Glucose tolerance test*	If clinical features of acromegaly present. Failure of growth hormone to suppress to unmeasurable levels confirms the diagnosis and this needs further investigation (**seek advice**).

diagnosis. Taking a detailed family history is crucial if MODY is suspected since, unlike type 1 diabetes, the condition has an autosomal dominant inheritance. There is considerable variation in clinical expression; most affected families have modest hyperglycaemia with a low risk of long-term microvascular complications. Approximately half the reported cases of MODY are due to abnormalities of the glucokinase gene causing impaired glucose sensing and insulin release from β-cells. MODY accounts for <1% of cases of "garden type" type 2 diabetes.

There are numerous genetic disorders associated with diabetes. All are rare but a few examples are shown in Box 1.2.

Long-term complications

This is an important question in a newly diagnosed type 2 patient because microvascular and macrovascular complications may be found at diagnosis (Table 1.3) and, if present, may require urgent assessment (see later chapters).

Table 1.3   Prevalence of long-term complications in diabetes[10]

Complication	Prevalence (%)
Retinopathy (at least one microaneurysm)	21
Abnormal ECG	18
Absent foot pulses (two or more)	14
Impaired reflexes and/or decreased vibration sense	7
Angina	3
Intermittent claudication	3
Myocardial infarction	2
Stroke/transient ischaemic attack	1

Based on the findings in the history and examination, a number of investigations will be needed. These can be classified as "essential", or "if clinically indicated" (Box 1.3).

References

1 World Health Organisation. *WHO Study Group on diabetes mellitus.* Technical Report Series 727. Geneva: WHO, 1985.
2 American Diabetes Association. Report on the diagnosis and classification of diabetes mellitus. *Diabetes Care* 1997;**20**:1183–97.

3 Molbak AG, Christau B, Marner B *et al.* Incidence of insulin-dependent diabetes in age groups over 30 years in Denmark. *Diabetic Med* 1994; **11**:650–5.

4 Olmos P, A'Hern R, Heaton DA *et al.* The significance of the concordance rate for Type-1 (insulin-dependent) diabetes in identical twins. *Diabetologia* 1988;**31**:747–50.

5 Thorsby E, Ronningen KS. Particular HLA-DQ molecules play a dominant role in determining susceptibility or resistance to Type-1 (insulin-dependent) diabetes mellitus. *Diabetologia* 1993;**36**:371–7.

6 Eisenbarth GS. Type-1 diabetes mellitus. A chronic autoimmune disease. *New Engl J Med* 1986;**314**:1360–8.

7 Yki-Jarvinen H. Pathogenesis of non-insulin-dependent diabetes mellitus. *Lancet* 1994;**343**:91–5.

8 Riddle MC. *Endocrinol Metab Clin N Amer* 1997;**26**:662.

9 Tattersall RB. Mild familial diabetes with dominant inheritance. *Q J Med* 1974;**43**:339–57.

10 United Kingdom Prospective Diabetes Study. *Diabetologia* 1991;**34**: 877–90.

2 Treatment of diabetes

Because 10% of hospital beds are occupied by people with diabetes, it is important that medical staff have a working knowledge of the available treatments, how they are used and what side effects may occur.

Insulin

Before the principles of insulin treatment are described, it is useful to know about the physiological secretion of insulin, since many of the common regimens attempt, with varying degrees of success, to mimic this profile.

Insulin physiology

Physiologically insulin is secreted in two phases (Figure 2.1):

- during fasting, secretion is at a constant "basal" rate, whilst
- after meals, insulin is rapidly secreted into the portal circulation providing a "post-prandial" peak to control the post-meal rise in blood sugar.

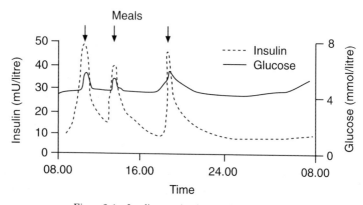

Figure 2.1 Insulin secretion in non-diabetic subjects.

Half the insulin is cleared with the first pass through the liver; the rest reaches the peripheral circulation where its action is regulated by rapid clearance with a half-life measured in minutes. This system is very sensitive and limits blood glucose increases after meals to no more than 1–2 mmol/litre.

Insulin types

A range of insulin preparations are available which are usually used in combination to match this physiological profile (Table 2.1).

Table 2.1   Examples of different insulin preparations

Insulin	Onset	Peak	Duration
Ultrashort-acting Lispro	10–20 min	30–60 min	3–4 hours
Short-acting Actrapid Velosulin Humulin S	30 min	1–3 hours	6–8 hours
Intermediate-acting Insulatard Humulin I Monotard	1–2 hours	4–8 hours	12–16 hours
Long-acting Humulin Zn Ultratard Bovine Lente Bovine PZI	3–4 hours	6–14 hours	24–30 hours

Ultrashort-acting (monomeric) insulins

The position of two amino acids has been reversed in insulin-Lispro so that, unlike soluble insulin, the molecules do not aggregate into hexamers. Lispro is therefore absorbed more quickly and has a shorter duration of action than soluble insulin. When given immediately before a meal, it controls post-prandial hyperglycaemia better than soluble insulin but, because of its shorter duration of action, blood glucose tends to rise before the next meal. It is often necessary to increase the basal insulin dose when people are transferred from soluble to Lispro insulin to compensate for this. These monomeric insulins work more rapidly than short-acting insulins.

Short-acting (soluble) insulin

Soluble insulin is manufactured using recombinant DNA technology and is highly purified. Subcutaneous injections of soluble insulin should be given 20–30 minutes before meals, unless the premeal blood sugar is low, when injection immediately before a meal is advisable. It is the only insulin preparation that should be used for intramuscular injection or intravenously in the treatment of ketoacidosis (Chapter 3) or perioperative management (Chapter 5).

Intermediate-acting insulin

The duration of action of insulin can be increased by mixing it with protamine and zinc to form Isophane (NPH) insulin, or with excess zinc forming Lente insulin. A striking feature of both preparations is the marked variability of absorption which can result in up to a 50% difference in blood insulin levels, even when the same dose is injected into the same site on successive injections. In clinical practice there is little to choose between the two preparations.[1]

Doses of intermediate-acting insulin should not be adjusted too often; this will avoid the knock-on effect from one day to the next. This is sometimes seen in hospital when staff may increase the dose every day, until the patient has a series of hypos (Chapter 4). It is more sensible to wait two or three days to see the full effect, before deciding whether further increases are needed. It is also worth emphasising that, because of the variation of absorption, increases of 1 or 2 units are unlikely to make much difference. When a patient has persistent hyperglycaemia, a 10% increase in the dose of intermediate insulin, divided between the daily injections is reasonable, with a further increase three days later if there has been no improvement.

Long-acting insulin

Current preparations such as Ultratard and Humulin Zn, although claiming a duration of over 24 hours, do not achieve this in practice. In fact, Humulin Zn can be used interchangeably with intermediate-acting insulin with no appreciable effect on control. Bovine insulins (Lente and PZI) are the longest acting insulins available. Bovine insulin is more antigenic than human insulin, and regular use stimulates antibodies which "bind" insulin in the circulation, thereby prolonging its duration of action.[2]

Species

Three species of insulin are available: bovine, porcine and human. *Bovine insulin* differs from human by three amino acids and *porcine insulin* by one. Switching between insulin species is not recommended because it can cause problems with control. This is particularly so when switching people from bovine to *human insulin*, and a reduction of 10–20% of the overall dose is usually needed when bovine insulin is switched to human insulin to avoid unexpected hypoglycaemia. Always specify both the species and type of insulin to be administered.

If a patient has been on bovine insulin for 40 years and is admitted to your ward, it is meddlesome (and will cause a lot of anger from the patient) to change them onto human insulin.

With the introduction of human insulin in the 1980s, many people with diabetes have been transferred from animal to human insulin, despite the lack of evidence of clinical benefit. As a result, demand for animal insulin is declining, but be aware that there is a small but vociferous minority who have tried human insulin, claim it reduces their warning of hypoglycaemia, and insist on animal insulin at all times. You should respect their wishes.

Commonly used insulin regimens

There remains an "air of mystery" about the use of insulin amongst many non-specialist doctors, who may be confused by the range of preparations, uncertain about how to "choose the right dose" and daunted by the consequences of "getting it wrong", precipitating hypoglycaemia or hyperglycaemia. In fact, the principles of insulin therapy are relatively straightforward and can be guided by a few simple "rules of thumb" (Box 2.1).

Starting regimen

People with newly diagnosed type 1 diabetes are usually started on human insulin, because it provides the widest choice of injection methods, including syringe and needle, pen injection devices and disposable pens. For a suitable starting regimen, the aims are:

- relief of symptoms;
- providing essential "first-aid" information for the first few days;
- keeping things simple;
- avoiding hypoglycaemia.

21

Box 2.1 Guidelines for insulin therapy

- Daily insulin requirements are usually 0.5–1 unit/kg (35–70 units for a 70 kg man).
- About two-thirds of total insulin production is basal, with one-third related to meals.
- People on twice daily injections usually take about two-thirds of their daily dose in the morning and one-third in the evening. One-third of the morning dose is usually short-acting and two-thirds intermediate-acting insulin. The evening dose is usually nearer 50:50 between short- and intermediate-acting insulin.
- People on a basal bolus regimen should take 30–40% of their total dose as medium-acting insulin before bed. The remainder should be given as soluble insulin in divided doses before meals, depending on meal size and amount of carbohydrate.
- Insulin requirements increase during intercurrent illness, pregnancy or steroid treatment, often with a two- to three-fold increase in total daily dose.

Twice daily intermediate-acting insulin, with injections given 30 minutes before breakfast and the evening meal, achieves these objectives.[3] Suitable starting doses are 6–10 units twice daily, and this should be increased every few days by 2–4 units until symptoms resolve and glycaemic control is stabilised. This is best judged by home blood glucose tests, which the patient should be taught to do one or two weeks after diagnosis. As blood glucose levels fall, remaining beta-cells recover, albeit temporarily, and insulin doses usually need to be reduced to avoid hypoglycaemia between six weeks and four months after diagnosis. Occasionally, people may be able to stop insulin altogether during the "honeymoon period", but some find having to restart, when blood sugars deteriorate, more difficult to accept. It is usually better to recommend continuing with small doses of insulin throughout this honeymoon period. When daily doses exceed 25–30 units, it is usually necessary to add short-acting insulin to control blood sugar after breakfast and the evening meal.

The time course of action of these regimens is illustrated in Figures 2.2–2.4.

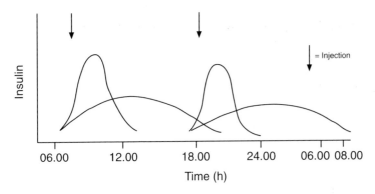

Figure 2.2   Time course of action of twice daily short- and intermediate-acting insulin.

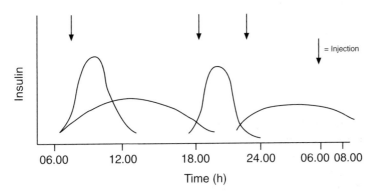

Figure 2.3   Time course of action of split-evening insulin.

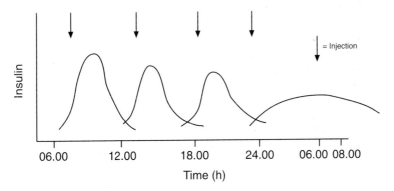

Figure 2.4   Time course of action of basal bolus regimen.

23

Twice daily short- and intermediate-acting insulin (Figure 2.2)

Advantages
- Simple, convenient and fits well into many people's workday routine.
- Premixed insulins available ranging from 10:90% short:intermediate to 50:50 short:intermediate. The most commonly used mixture is 30:70.

Disadvantages
- Limited flexibility with the timing of meals. A delayed lunch may result in hypoglycaemia.
- Overnight blood sugar control can be a problem, especially if the main evening meal is eaten at 5.00 pm, with a risk of hypoglycaemia in the early hours of the morning, and hyperglycaemia on waking because of declining insulin levels.

Split-evening insulin (Figure 2.3)

Advantages
- Better control of morning glucose.
- Less risk of overnight hypoglycaemia.

Disadvantages
- Limited flexibility with daytime meals. A delayed lunch may result in hypoglycaemia.
- Three injections rather than two.

Basal bolus regimen (Figure 2.4)

Advantages
- More flexibility with meal times.
- Able to vary meal size and give appropriate insulin dose.

Disadvantages
- Four injections
- Flexibility with meal size can lead to weight gain of, on average, 2–3 kg.

Special groups

Children

Infants and small children are usually managed on a simple regimen of once daily intermediate-acting insulin, which is associated with a low risk of hypoglycaemia. In older children (usually from about 8 years of age), twice daily regimens using short- and intermediate-acting insulins are needed to control diabetes, and such regimens fit well with school hours. Regimens are usually continued during early adolescence, but multiple injection regimens may be introduced at this stage when greater flexibility is needed.

Pregnancy

Pregnancy is associated with insulin resistance, particularly from the end of the second trimester to term, as a result of the effects of placental hormones. In non-diabetic women, this resistance is automatically overcome by compensatory hyperinsulinaemia, but those with type 1 diabetes must adjust (usually increase) their insulin doses frequently to achieve the normal blood sugars associated with the best outcome for the child. A multiple injection regimen of soluble insulin before meals, and bedtime isophane or lente insulin offers the greatest flexibility, although a few women continue to use twice daily injections of premixed insulin.

Total daily doses of insulin three or more times higher than before conception are often needed to maintain glucose control in the third trimester. Insulin sensitivity returns to normal within hours after delivery of the placenta, and insulin requirements return to preconception levels. It is useful to have a record of the daily preconception insulin dose, since it can sometimes be a difficult figure for the mother to remember.

The elderly

Many elderly people with diabetes are able to manage twice daily injection regimens, particularly with the convenience offered by pen-injection devices. Problems can arise with increasing frailty, deteriorating mental ability or poor vision, all of which make accurate insulin administration more difficult. Sometimes, family are available who can be shown how to administer insulin twice daily. An alternative is transferring to a once daily insulin regimen, which can then be supervised by a district nurse. Bovine lente insulin is one such option, with the dose adjusted to achieve a fasting blood glucose, measured by the district nurse, of 7–11 mmol/litre.

Type 2 diabetes

Oral hypoglycaemic drugs are used in about two-thirds of people with type 2 diabetes. Their use should always be seen as an adjunct to diet, which should form the cornerstone of management.

Diet

People need a simple explanation of what diabetes is, how high blood sugar levels cause symptoms and the effect that meals have on blood sugar. The importance of the link between diet and blood sugar should be emphasised, so that the need for dietary change is understood.

Modern diabetic diets are similar to those for "healthy eating" in the general population, with an emphasis on limiting intake of refined carbohydrate (sugars) and saturated fat, and reducing total energy intake by overweight patients. Complex carbohydrates (starchy foods) have less effect on blood glucose than refined sugars, and should provide 50–60% of energy intake.

Initial dietary advice is best given on a one-to-one basis by a dietitian, supported by written information and reinforced at follow-up appointments. Group education sessions held within a few weeks of diagnosis can help people to share experiences, and provide the opportunity for other aspects of diabetic care to be covered.

Three further points about dietary advice should be made:

- It is important when a diet plan is being designed to take a careful history of the person's current eating habits, including likes and dislikes. Success is more likely if recommendations are based on modest changes rather than attempting a complete overhaul.
- It is useful to provide a target weight, although this has to be realistic. There is little point in telling someone whose weight has been stable at 16 stone (224 lb) for 20 years that the ideal target weight should be no higher than 11 stone (144 lb)!

- A weight loss of 0.5–1 kg/week is ideal; "crash" or very low calorie diets should be avoided. Sustaining a long-term change in eating habits to maintain a normal weight should be stressed.

The success of any diet is measured by its effect on symptoms, weight and blood glucose control. Fasting glucose provides a simple, reproducible and inexpensive way of monitoring glycaemic response to diet, and should be measured two or three times in the first three months.

Current European guidelines suggest that a fasting blood glucose of <7.8 mmol/litre is "borderline" and 4.4–6.1 mmol/litre "good".[4] These levels are not set in stone and may be inappropriate for some people. Individual glycaemic targets should take into account age, social circumstances (e.g. it is desirable for a person living alone to have a low risk of hypoglycaemia), mental state, associated medical conditions and extent of diabetic complications.

Sulphonylureas

These drugs work mainly by stimulating insulin secretion from beta-cells, but they also reduce insulin resistance to some extent.[5] Commonly available preparations are listed in Table 2.2.

Table 2.2   Characteristics of various sulphonylurea drugs

Sulphonylurea	Dose/day	Half life (h)	Dose regimen	Active metabolite	Renal clearance (%)
Tolbutamide	1.0–3.0 g	3–8	Divided	+	100
Chlorpropamide	50–500 mg	35	Single daily	+	100
Glibenclamide	2.5–20 mg	5	Single or divided	±	50
Glipizide	1.25–20 mg	4	Single or divided	−	85
Gliclazide	40–320 mg	12	Single or divided	−	60

The lowest possible dose should be used initially with increases every two to four weeks until adequate glycaemic control is achieved.

Occasionally, sulphonylureas do not work from the outset (primary failure of therapy) because people may have type 1 diabetes or LADA. Secondary sulphonylurea failure, where glycaemic control gradually deteriorates with time despite progressive increases in dose, may result from non-compliance with diet, but usually reflects the progressive decline in beta-cell

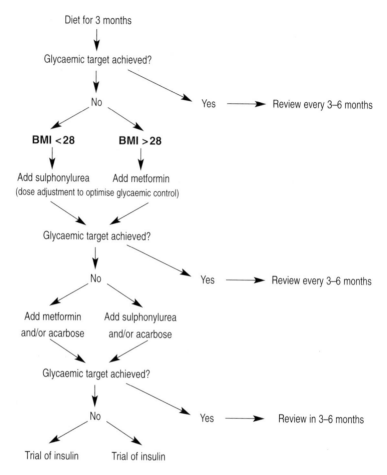

Figure 2.5 Protocol for managing hyperglycaemia in type 2 diabetes.

function. It is a common problem and some have even suggested that all patients on tablets will not respond after 10 years.

Any sulphonylurea will cause weight gain if a person continues to overeat. By lowering blood glucose, sulphonylureas (and insulin) reduce the leak of calories into the urine, with the result that patients tend to gain weight if they continue with their usual diet. In clinical trials, this averages about 2 kg, but some people may gain 10 kg or more, which may offset any benefit of the drug.

Starting a sulphonylurea is not a substitute for dietary compliance. Because of this weight gain, sulphonylureas should not be used as first-line drugs in overweight patients.

The major side effect of sulphonylureas is hypoglycaemia (see Chapter 4), and minor episodes may occur in 20% of patients on treatment.[6] People should be told about the typical symptoms and what to do if they occur. The elderly are particularly vulnerable, especially if long-acting drugs, such as chlorpropamide or glibenclamide, are used.[7] These should be avoided in patients >70 years of age.

Other side effects are rare and confined to particular preparations. If used in high doses (>500 mg) chlorpropamide occasionally causes reversible cholestatic jaundice, and may also cause dilutional hyponatraemia because of an antidiuretic effect on the kidney. Transient flushing following alcohol can occur in up to 25% of people on chlorpropamide, and in all those where the serum chlorpropamide level is high enough.

Biguanides

Metformin, a biguanide, is often used as first-line therapy in overweight people because it does not cause weight gain. It has been used in Europe since 1959 and has recently been licensed in North America. It inhibits glucose production from the liver and enhances peripheral glucose uptake by skeletal muscle.[8] Unlike sulphonylureas, it does not stimulate insulin and has no risk of hypoglycaemia although, when used in combination with a sulphonylurea, the hypoglycaemic effects of the latter are increased. Metformin is excreted unchanged through the kidneys. The therapeutic dose is 1–3 g/day in divided doses.

Gastrointestinal side effects, including nausea, abdominal pain and diarrhoea, occur in up to 25% of those on metformin and are dose-dependent. They can be minimised by starting with a low dose and increasing at weekly intervals. Those unfamiliar with such side effects may embark on extensive, but unnecessary, gastrointestinal investigations, including barium studies and endoscopies, in someone presenting with a "change of bowel habit". It is always worth stopping metformin to see if the symptoms go away before going down this route of investigation. A few patients are unable to tolerate metformin even at 1 g/day without gastrointestinal side effects.

The major side effect associated with metformin is lactic acidosis. Over 100 cases have been reported worldwide and, in the vast majority, it develops in association with chronic renal failure as a result of reduced renal clearance of metformin. Metformin should not be used in those whose plasma creatinine is >150 μmol/litre.

Lactic acidosis can also occur in patients with acute heart failure, owing to a combination of tissue hypoxia from reduced cardiac output together with reduced excretion of metformin from renal hypoperfusion. Metformin should be stopped in those presenting with heart failure or myocardial infarction, and alternative methods should be used to control hyperglycaemia (see Chapter 3). People with stable heart failure are at much lower risk and metformin can be continued, provided the left ventricular function is not grossly impaired.

A recent recommendation from the UK Royal College of Radiologists, based on the manufacturer's data sheet, states that, to avoid any risk of lactic acidosis, metformin should be stopped for 48 hours before radiological procedures that use intravenous contrast medium. The risks are extremely small, but radiology departments in the UK are required to adopt these guidelines, and it is important to advise patients accordingly to avoid unnecessary postponement of investigations.

Alpha-glucosidase inhibitors

These drugs irreversibly bind to the glucosidase enzyme of the intestinal brush border. *Acarbose* is the only agent available in the UK, but others are available worldwide. They delay the absorption of glucose from the intestine resulting in a smaller rise of blood glucose after meals. Post-prandial insulin responses are also lower, and there is a modest effect on overall glycaemic control.[9]

The main side effects of flatus and diarrhoea result from fermentation of unabsorbed carbohydrate in the large bowel. This can be reduced by starting with low doses and increasing slowly over two to three months, but even then up to 50% of patients remain intolerant.

Alpha-glucosidase inhibitors do not cause hypoglycaemia themselves but, when used in combination with sulphonylureas, they make the treatment of hypoglycaemia more difficult, because oral sucrose (sugar) will be ineffective. People taking this combination of tablets should be provided with glucose tablets (Dextrosol) to treat the hypoglycaemia.

Thiazolidinediones

The thiazolidinediones are a new class of oral antidiabetic agent; they act as "insulin sensitisers". They lower blood glucose without stimulating insulin secretion and, typically, endogenous insulin levels fall during treatment.[10] *Troglitazone*, the only thiazolidinedione currently available (not in the UK) has similar hypoglycaemic potency to the sulphonylureas and metformin, although about 20% of patients do not respond. Non-responders tend to be those with marked insulin deficiency, suggesting that the drug requires adequate insulin levels for its hypoglycaemic properties to be manifest.

Troglitazone is currently only available in America and Japan. It was launched in the UK in late 1997, but supply was suspended after six weeks following reports of hepatotoxicity in other countries. Several deaths due to irreversible hepatic failure have occurred on treatment, although a direct causal relationship with troglitazone remains to be established. Several other thiazolidinediones are likely to become available in the near future.

Protocol for the management of hyperglycaemia in type 2 diabetes

Evidence-based medical practice has been difficult to apply to type 2 diabetes because evidence from long-term clinical trials has, until recently, been unavailable. The United Kingdom Prospective Diabetes Study (UKPDS)[11,12] has now provided clear evidence of benefit in treating blood glucose (and blood pressure) in type 2 diabetes. The UKPDS compared diet, sulphonylureas, metformin, acarbose or insulin in the treatment of over 5000 patients with newly diagnosed type 2 diabetes to determine, first, whether intensive glucose control lowered the risk of long-term complications and, second, whether any of the available drugs had advantages or disadvantages. A summary of the key findings is shown in Table 2.3.

31

Table 2.3 Summary of key findings in the UKPDS glucose control study

Intensive glucose control (mean HBA$_{1c}$ 7.0%) lowered		*P*
● All diabetes-related complications	12%	0.029
● Myocardial infarction	16%	0.052
● Microvascular complications	25%	0.0099
Metformin in overweight patients lowered		
● All diabetes-related complications	32%	0.0023
● Diabetes-related deaths	42%	0.017
● All cause mortality	36%	0.011
● Myocardial infarction	39%	0.01
Treatment groups		
● No difference in clinical endpoint incidence between glibenclamide, chlorpropamide and insulin		
● Weight gain and hypoglycaemia significantly higher for sulphonylurea and insulin compared with diet alone or metformin		

The UKPDS results support an intensive approach to management of blood glucose in patients diagnosed under 65 years of age to minimise the long-term risk of microvascular complications. This is best assessed using the HBA$_{1c}$, a measure of non-enzymatic glycation of haemoglobin which correlates with average blood glucose concentrations over the six to eight weeks before the sample is taken. A target of 7% or less is ideal. Most patients will need medication in addition to diet to achieve this and, given the similar efficacy of sulphonylureas and insulin, it is sensible to start normal weight patients on a sulphonylurea and switch them to insulin, if glycaemic targets are no longer met as the disease progresses. Metformin has clear advantages in overweight patients and should be used as first-line therapy.

Another message from the UKPDS is that, in view of the benefits of maintaining long-term tight glycaemic control, a trial of insulin should no longer be considered as the therapeutic equivalent of the "end of the road", but considered as soon as diet and tablets no longer achieve the glycaemic target. A protocol for managing hyperglycaemia in type 2 diabetes is shown in Figure 2.5.

It is important to emphasise that glycaemic targets should be individualised. In the UKPDS the benefits of tight glycaemic control took almost a decade to become apparent, and this should be borne in mind when suitable glycaemic targets for elderly patients are being discussed, for whom symptom control and avoidance of hypoglycaemia are the prime management objectives.

Insulin in type 2 diabetes

Overall, 20% of patients with type 2 diabetes need insulin to control hyperglycaemia. The longer patients have had diabetes, the greater the likelihood that they will need insulin to control hyperglycaemia; at 15 years the proportion rises to 50%. The link with disease duration also accounts for the greater likelihood of microvascular complications in those patients on insulin than in those on diet or tablets alone.

Doctors (and patients) are often reluctant to recommend insulin in type 2 diabetes. Patients fear injections or believe that insulin is in some way addictive and, once started, can never be stopped. Others think that insulin treatment means that their diabetes is more serious. Doctors are concerned about weight gain or the risk of hypoglycaemia in elderly patients. However, the results of the UKPDS provide clear evidence of the benefits of intensive glucose control with either sulphonylureas or insulin, and it is likely that, in the future, more patients will be switched to insulin to maintain optimal glycaemic targets.

Clinical experience suggests that most normal weight patients, whose diabetes results more from relative insulin deficiency than insulin resistance, eventually need insulin therapy and feel better for it. The benefit in overweight patients is harder to predict, but over half will feel better on insulin, even if their diabetic control is unchanged. In patients with obvious symptoms of hyperglycaemia, despite diet and tablets, the decision to switch to insulin is usually straightforward. It is more difficult in those who claim to feel well but in whom diabetic control remains poor. A therapeutic trial is a sensible option under these circumstances, since some people only realise after starting insulin that they had been experiencing symptoms. Most should achieve better diabetic control on insulin, usually of the order of a 2% fall in HBA_{1c} concentrations.[13] The decision to recommend a trial of insulin must take into account symptoms, age, complications, family support and implications for employment. There is little point in browbeating a reluctant patient, but fears about the injection itself can often be allayed by a dummy injection in the clinic. It is also worth agreeing with the patient that if, after a three-month trial of insulin, they feel no better, they can return to tablets. The principles of insulin treatment in type 2 diabetes are similar to those in type 1, but regimens tend to be simpler (Box 2.2).

Weight gain is a common problem on insulin and is mainly due to the preservation of energy that was previously lost through glycosuria. Most trials report average increases of 2–4 kg, but some patients may gain 10 kg or more. The insulin regimen used has little effect on the degree of weight gain and it is important to reinforce dietary principles, preferably with the help of a dietician beforehand.

Combination therapy with sulphonylureas and insulin is more popular in some countries than others. Tablets are taken during the day with a bedtime injection of isophane or lente insulin. The rationale is that controlling fasting blood glucose with bedtime insulin will reduce "glucotoxicity" so that the sulphonylurea controls post-prandial glucose excursions. Sulphonylureas can, therefore, be thought of as providing an "insulin-sparing" effect, but there is no evidence that such regimens are better than insulin alone. When twice daily insulin becomes necessary to maintain control, most diabetologists recommend insulin by itself, to avoid the inconvenience of taking injections and tablets. One exception to this general rule is the combination of metformin and insulin. In overweight people and those who need insulin to improve glycaemic control, a combination with metformin can help to limit the weight-promoting consequences of a trial of insulin.[14]

Box 2.2 Guidelines for insulin therapy in type 2 diabetes

- Most patients should start on twice daily premixed short- and intermediate-acting insulin.
- A convenient starting dose is 0.3–0.4 unit/kg/day, with two-thirds of the dose given before breakfast and one-third before the evening meal.
- A comprehensive education programme is needed, as for people with type 1 diabetes.
- Frequent review by a diabetes specialist nurse and dietitian is needed to deal with problems.
- Review diabetic control, weight, diet and sense of well-being after three months.

Managing diabetes in hospital

People with diabetes account for about 10% of the inpatient workload of general hospitals in most developed countries. A minority will be hospitalised because of poor glycaemic control, as either hyper- or hypoglycaemia, and management of these problems is discussed in Chapters 3 and 4. Most will be admitted for a diabetes-related complication or treatment of an unrelated condition. An important part of their care should include an assessment of diabetic control and complications.

A comprehensive history should include:

- the duration and type of diabetes
- current treatment(s)
- self-monitoring (urinalysis or self measured blood glucose)
- problems with control
- extent of supervision in primary care or hospital clinics
- history of microvascular or macrovascular complications and their treatment
- whether eye screening has been regular to detect sight-threatening retinopathy (patients who have not had an eye examination within the last year should be assessed (see Chapter 9))
- blood pressure measurement
- urine test for protein

These assessments help to determine the extent to which diabetes will influence other aspects of clinical management.

How well controlled should diabetes be?

A hospital ward is a difficult place to achieve good diabetic control. Diet and day-to-day activities will be very different from usual, and intercurrent illness may cause significant counter-regulatory hormone responses that will increase insulin needs. People may need to fast to prepare for investigations or surgery.

The biggest problem is that no one person is in control. Nominally the house physician or house surgeon should be, but he or she is usually inexperienced and does not have time or confidence to change insulin doses before each meal. Each patient should have a named nurse but, even if they do in practice, the nurse does not have the authority to change insulin doses. There is also subtle pressure exerted by the nurses on the house physician

35

to avoid hypos at all costs, since these are seen as a failure and upset the other patients. The failure of sliding scales is considered below.

When patients are admitted with an intercurrent illness, such as infection, or for surgery, it seems clinically prudent to aim for near normoglycaemia during the admission. It has been suggested that this may improve neutrophil function and wound healing, although there is only evidence from trials in animals to support this. Occasionally, patients with newly diagnosed diabetes are admitted and, in this situation, achieving tight glycaemic control is not necessary—it may be associated with an increased risk of hypoglycaemia after discharge when the person is more active. It is more sensible to aim for moderate glycaemic control (blood glucose <15 mmol/litre) and to arrange for follow-up by the diabetes team soon after discharge.

Hyperglycaemic and hypoglycaemic emergencies, myocardial infarction and surgery are discussed in later chapters, but it is worth making some general points about in-hospital diabetic management and highlighting some commonly encountered clinical situations.

Poor control in type 2 diabetes

Many patients with type 2 diabetes are poorly controlled at home. When they get into hospital, there may be a temptation to adjust their dose of tablets. This will not improve diabetic control very quickly, because new steady-state drug concentrations take time to achieve—about a week for the longer acting sulphonylureas. If rapid control of blood glucose is necessary, for example in a preoperative workup, switching to insulin is usually the best option.

If rapid control is not necessary, an appropriate plan should be made depending on the cause of the poor control and whether the patient has hyperglycaemic symptoms. This may involve referral to a dietitian for advice and education, adjustment of tablets or switching to insulin with referral to the primary care physician or hospital specialist for further assessment.

Why subcutaneous sliding scales are not the answer for poor diabetic control

People with diabetes are often put on sliding scales when their blood glucoses are, or are likely to become, unstable. The dose of

Table 2.4 Intravenous insulin sliding scale

Capillary blood glucose (mmol/l)	Insulin infusion rate
0–3.9	0.5 units/h
4.0–6.9	1.0 units/h
7.0–9.9	2.0 units/h
10.0–14.9	3.0 units/h
≥ 15.0	4.0 mmol/litre

insulin is determined by the capillary blood glucose test, usually taken by the duty nurse immediately before each injection. Unfortunately all subcutaneous sliding scales are inherently illogical because, as someone has said, "You can't control diabetes backwards." The inevitable consequence is "roller coaster" blood glucose control with too much insulin being given when the blood glucose is high, and too little when it is low. A recent American study of 171 adults admitted with diabetes as a co-morbid condition found that sliding scales were associated with a three-fold increase in episodes of hyperglycaemia, compared with regimens that included a standing dose of intermediate-acting insulin.[15]

If the subcutaneous insulin sliding scale should not be used, what is the alternative? In patients who are unwell with unstable glycaemic control, an intravenous sliding scale with one to two hourly blood glucose testing is the best option. In theory, intravenous sliding scales work much better than subcutaneous ones because of the short half-life (minutes) of intravenous insulin, which allows "hour-by-hour" control of blood glucose. Average insulin requirements are about 40 units/day for a 70 kg patient with type 1 diabetes, and most sliding scales should aim to deliver 1 or 2 units/h (24–48 units/day), with blood glucose results in the range 4–10 mmol/litre. A typical sliding scale is shown in Table 2.4.

Intravenous sliding scales are by no means infallible. For example, we have seen one on a surgical ward which read:

Blood glucose	Insulin
<7	0
7–17	1 units/h
17–24	2 units/h

This led to a patient, admitted for a minor operation, developing ketoacidosis. Other ways in which an intravenous sliding scale can fail are:

- if blood glucose levels are misread by eye;
- if the pump is turned off—because the patient has no depot this immediately makes them insulin-deficient;
- if the pump is not connected to the patient.

When insulin is combined with an infusion of 5 or 10% dextrose plus potassium, *intravenous* sliding scales are ideal for optimising glycaemic control in patients, who are unable to have their normal meals because of illness. They are also ideal for the treatment of ketoacidosis and hyperosmolar non-ketotic coma (see Chapter 3), and for perioperative glucose control in surgery (see Chapter 5).

In patients who do not need an intravenous sliding scale, it is more logical to use a prescribed insulin regimen, with regular monitoring of blood glucose tests and adjustment of insulin doses. Patients already on insulin should maintain their usual injection regimen if possible, although it is sometimes necessary to switch from twice daily to basal bolus system. Additional "top-up" doses of soluble insulin can be given if the blood glucose is unacceptably high but, if this is necessary, the prescribed insulin regimen should be increased the following day to reflect the extra insulin requirements.

Finally, a word of caution about adjusting insulin doses, particularly in people who have had diabetes for a long time and who have a good understanding of their disease. The emphasis of modern diabetes management is to encourage self-adjustment of insulin on the basis of home blood glucose testing. It can be frustrating and sometimes frightening for people to have their diabetes "taken over" in the hospital, with insulin adjustments imposed upon them without discussion. In many instances patients can look after their own diabetes during a hospital admission, often very effectively. This should be encouraged. If control is poor, this is an ideal opportunity for re-education.

Switching from intravenous insulin

In patients with type 1 diabetes, the most sensible time to switch from intravenous to subcutaneous insulin is at the usual time of insulin administration, before a meal. Where there have been problems with eating, it is sensible to delay transfer until the patient can tolerate solid food and, since staffing levels are usually highest during the day, switching around breakfast is an ideal time. Patients with known type 1 diabetes will become severely insulin-deficient within minutes of their infusion being switched off because of the short half-life of intravenous insulin. It is usual, therefore, to continue the infusion of insulin for about one hour after the subcutaneous insulin and meal have been given, to allow time for the subcutaneous insulin to be absorbed.

Steroid treatment

The case history describes problems encountered with steroids in a person with diabetes.

Case Study 4

A 41-year-old Asian man was referred to hospital with typical symptoms of diabetes which had developed over the previous week. He had a history of asthma, treated with inhaled beta-agonists. He had presented to his general practitioner one week previously, complaining of shortness of breath and wheezing. He was prescribed 40 mg oral prednisolone and increased doses of beta-agonist. He developed thirst and polyuria two days later.

On admission his peak flow was improving (250 litres/min from 190 litres/min previously), and there were scattered wheezes in the chest. Blood glucose was markedly raised at 36 mmol/litre. Urea and electrolytes were normal and there was no ketonuria. He was started on an intravenous insulin sliding scale which controlled his hyperglycaemia, and his steroid dose was halved; inhaled steroids were introduced. The steroids were stopped two days later, and the blood sugar level settled in the range of 9–13 mmol/litre on diet alone. He received advice on diet and urinalysis and was discharged. At follow-up his diabetic symptoms had resolved, and his urinalysis was consistently negative. A 75 g oral glucose tolerance test was consistent with impaired glucose tolerance rather than diabetes.

In pharmacological doses, glucocorticoids increase insulin resistance, worsen diabetic control in people with diabetes and, as in the case described, precipitate clinical diabetes in patients with "latent" diabetes.[16] Dexamethasone, used in the treatment of cerebral oedema, is the most potent glucocorticoid, being 30 times more potent than hydrocortisone. Prednisolone is about five times as potent.

Glucocorticoids typically cause a small rise in fasting blood glucose, with marked increases in post-prandial glycaemia. People with poorly controlled type 2 diabetes have higher fasting glucose concentrations and may develop severe hyperglycaemia with steroids; transfer to insulin is usually necessary to maintain diabetic control. In people with biochemically less severe type 2 diabetes, oral hypoglycaemic drugs are usually needed, because diet alone usually does not work unless the steroid dose can be rapidly tailed off. In those with type 1 diabetes, significant increases in insulin dose are usually required according to the results of regular glucose monitoring.

The hyperglycaemic effects are temporary and dose-related; insulin or tablet doses need to be reduced gradually in line with the steroid dose. Newly diagnosed steroid-induced diabetes usually resolves once the steroids are stopped.

Glucocorticoids are sometimes given as a high-dose pulsed regimen over three to five days. A sliding-scale intravenous insulin regimen is the most appropriate way of controlling hyper-glycaemia with this treatment. It is usually necessary to use higher insulin infusion rates; doubling the rates shown in table 2.4 would be a good starting point.

Parenteral nutrition

Total parenteral nutrition (TPN) is used in the treatment of "bowel failure" irrespective of the cause. It is used in patients who are malnourished and severely ill and in whom there is usually increased insulin resistance from the stress response to the illness. As a result, hyperglycaemia can develop during TPN in people with no past history of diabetes, and it usually becomes more severe in those with diabetes. In all cases, hyperglycaemia should be controlled with intravenous insulin. This can be achieved by adding insulin to the TPN feed or by using a separate insulin infusion together with a sliding scale. The sliding-scale option is preferable in the acute situation when daily requirements are uncertain and the TPN feed rate is being increased, as this avoids the need to replace TPN feed bags if the added dose of insulin has proved incorrect.[17] With a sliding scale, daily requirements can be calculated from the total dose infused over the previous 24 hours, and it is possible to begin adding an appropriate dose of insulin to TPN feed bags once daily requirements are known.

Ward-based monitoring of diabetic control

Electronic meters are widely available in hospital wards for near-patient testing and, when used correctly, they provide accurate capillary glucose measurement from around 1.5 mmol/litre to 27–33 mmol/litre. Correct technique is the single most important factor in obtaining an accurate reading, and many studies have shown that both patients and nurses can produce inaccurate results in up to 50% of tests. A training programme is essential to ensure high quality testing; it is important that medical and nursing staff are familiar with the system in their hospital.

A number of case reports have highlighted how inaccurate or misleading blood glucose test results can influence management.

Case Study 5[18]

A 70-year-old female known with diabetes fell and dislocated her hip. On admission she was distressed and difficult to assess. A BM strip (read by eye) was 13 mmol/litre. She was given pethidine and was in the anaesthetic room awaiting operation when the laboratory blood sugar result of 45 mmol/litre was received. Further investigation confirmed ketoacidosis.

Table 2.5   Factors affecting the accuracy of capillary blood test results

Factor	Comment
Inaccurate meter code	Check correct strips and pack code number is inserted into meter
Haematocrit	Glucose measurements are falsely increased in anaemia and depressed in polycythaemia; caution in paediatric/neonatal special care baby units
Acidosis	Tends to underread in severe acidosis; caution in diabetic ketoacidois
Glucose concentration	Gross hyperglycaemia as seen with hyperosmolar non-ketotic coma can be underestimated
Hypoglycaemia	Less accurate in the hypoglycaemic range; always interpret the result in light of the patient's condition

Case Study 6[18]

A 72-year-old man, not known to be diabetic, collapsed at home after three days' malaise. He was drowsy, dehydrated and tender abdominally. BM strips read 10 and 13 mmol/litre. Laboratory tests, performed only after urinalysis had shown heavy glycosuria, showed 80.4 mmol/litre glucose and a hyperosmolar state.

Several factors can affect the accuracy of capillary blood test results (Table 2.5) particularly in ill patients. The clinical message

Table 2.6   Frequency of glucose monitoring

Diabetes	Patient's condition	
	"Well"	"Ill"
Type 1	Pre-meal and pre-bedtime	1–2 hourly with sliding scale
Type 2	Fasting and post-prandial urinalysis Occasional fasting glucose	Pre-meal and pre-bedtime 1–2 hourly with sliding scale

---

Box 2.3 Questions to ask when faced with unknown patient with raised blood glucose

- *Is it type 1 or type 2 diabetes?* Patients with type 1 diabetes often have marked changes in blood glucose and these levels may swing from >20 to <4 mmol/litre in the space of a few hours. Those with type 2 diabetes have more predictable fasting and post-prandial blood glucose levels

- *Is the patient unwell?* A blood glucose of 24.5 mmol/litre is of less concern if the patient is up and about, is not vomiting and does not have ketonuria

- *Is there a pattern?* Are other results available, to look for a pattern of change? Are they always high at this time or is this a "one off" result?

- *Are there ketones?* If present, this would suggest the need for more insulin in those with type 1, and for starting insulin in those with type 2 diabetes

- *Does the patient think there is a problem?* Patients with type 1 diabetes often know their diabetes best. It is worth asking what they would do with this result if they were at home

Box 2.4 Management guidelines for a hospital patient with diabetes

Diabetes	If the patient is well (up and about, no ketones)	If the patient is ill (especially with ketonuria)
Type 1 Blood glucose of 15–20 mmol/litre	Repeat test in 2–4 hours; look for a pattern in previous tests; if usually high at this time, adjust appropriate insulin dose	Give 6–10 units **soluble** insulin and repeat 4 hours later; monitor urinary ketones; may need intravenous insulin sliding scale
Blood glucose >20 mmol/litre	Give 6–10 units of soluble insulin s.c. and repeat 4 hours later; if usually high at this time, adjust appropriate insulin dose	Intravenous insulin sliding scale especially if patient has nausea and vomiting, or urinary ketones
Type 2 Blood glucose of 15–20 mmol/litre	Review diet for compliance; review previous results; adjust dose of oral hypoglycaemic drugs if consistent finding	Adjust oral hypolgycaemic dose if possible; consider (temporary) transfer to insulin, especially if intercurrent illness present
Blood glucose >20 mmol/litre	Review diet and oral hypoglycaemic drugs; check urine for ketones; may need insulin if persistent and no precipitant	Give 6–10 units **soluble** insulin s.c. and repeat 4 hours later; monitor urinary ketones; may need (temporary) transfer to insulin, either with fixed doses or intravenous sliding scale

is that the result of capillary blood tests should always be interpreted in the light of the patient's clinical condition, and should always be confirmed with laboratory measurements in emergency situations.

Frequency of testing

The intensity of monitoring of blood or urine glucose testing should be tailored to the clinical situation; obviously a patient with type 1 diabetes admitted with pneumonia will require more frequent testing than a patient with diet-controlled type 2 diabetes admitted electively for a laparoscopic cholecystectomy. Many patients are monitored with capillary blood tests before meals and bedtime, irrespective of their type of diabetes and level of control. This is unnecessary and wasteful, particularly in patients with type 2 diabetes who are reasonably well controlled, since their day-to-day fluctuations of blood glucose are reproducible. Such patients can be more appropriately monitored with urinalysis, with occasional fasting capillary glucose measurements.

A suggested frequency for glucose monitoring for types 1 and 2 diabetes is shown in Table 2.6. This should be reviewed regularly to avoid unnecessary tests being done simply as a routine.

Capillary blood glucose testing often raises questions for medical staff. A typical scenario is for the on-call doctor to be faced with a patient (usually unknown to them) with a blood glucose of 24.5 mmol/litre, for example, and the nurse in charge asking, "What should be done?" All too often this results in a prescription for anywhere between 2 and 10 units of short-acting insulin without a full assessment of the problem. The questions in Box 2.3 may help in deciding what to do.

Management guidelines for dealing with this common scenario are provided in Box 2.4.

References

1 Tunbridge FKE, Newens A, Home PD *et al.* Double-blind cross-over trial of isophane (NPH) and lente-based insulin regimens. *Diabetes Care* 1989;**12**:115–19.
2 Hildebrandt P, Berger A, Volund A, Kuhl C. The subcutaneous absorption of human and bovine ultralente insulin. *Diabetic Med* 1985; **2**:355–9.
3 Wilson RM, Clarke P, Bailes H, Heller S, Tattersall RB. Initiation of insulin treatment as an outpatient. *J Am Med Ass* 1986;**256**:877–80.

4 Alberti KGMM, Gries FA, Jeruell J, Krans HMJ. A desktop guide for the management of non-insulin-dependent diabetes mellitus (NIDDM): an update. *Diabetic Med.* 1994;**11**:899–909.

5 Groop L. Sulphonylureas in NIDDM. *Diabetes Care* 1992;**15**:737–54.

6 Jennings AM, Wilson RM, Ward JD. Symptomatic hypoglycaemia in NIDDM patients treated with oral hypoglycaemic agents. *Diabetes Care* 1989;**12**:203–8.

7 Asplund K, Wiholm B-E, Lithner F. Glibenclamide associated hypoglycaemia: a report of 57 cases. *Diabetologia* 1983;**24**:412.

8 Bailey CJ. Biguanides and NIDDM. *Diabetes Care* 1992;**15**:755–72.

9 Chaisson JL, Josse RG, Hunt JA *et al*. The efficacy of acarbose in the treatment of patients with non-insulin-dependent diabetes mellitus. *Ann Intern Med* 1994;**121**:928–35.

10 Kumar S, Boulton AJ, Beck-Neilsen H *et al*. Troglitazone, an insulin enhancer, improves metabolic control in NIDDM patients. *Diabetologia* 1996;**39**:701–9.

11 United Kingdom Prospective Diabetes Study, 33. Intensive blood-glucose control with sulphonylureas or insulin compared with conventional treatment and risk of complications in patients with type 2 diabetes. *Lancet* 1998;**352**:837–53.

12 United Kingdom Prospective Diabetes Study, 34. Effect of intensive blood-glucose control with metformin on complications in overweight patients with type 2 diabetes. *Lancet* 1998;**352**:854–65.

13 Yki-Jarvinen H, Kaupplia M, Kujansuu E *et al*. Comparison of insulin regimens in patients with non-insulin-dependent diabetes. *New Engl J Med* 1992;**327**:1426–33.

14 Yki-Jarvinen H, Ryysy L, Nikkila K *et al*. Comparison of bedtime insulin regimens in patient with type 2 diabetes mellitus. *Ann Intern Med* 1999;**130**:389–96.

15 Queale WS, Seidler AJ, Brancati FL. Glycaemic control and sliding scale insulin use in medical inpatients with diabetes mellitus. *Arch Intern Med* 1997;**157**:545–52.

16 Hirsch IB, Paauw DS. Diabetes management in special situations. *Endocrinol Metab Clin N Amer* 1997;**26**:631–45.

17 Sajbel TA, Dutro MP, Radway PR. Use of separate insulin infusions with total parenteral nutrition. *J Parenteral Enteral Nutr* 1987;**11**: 97–100.

18 Coppack SW, Mitchell D, McIntosh CS. Accuracy of BM test glycemic 20–800 strips. *Diabetic Med* 1985;**3**:146.

3 Hyperglycaemic diabetic emergencies

There are two forms of hyperglycaemic diabetic emergency: diabetic ketoacidosis (DKA) and hyperosmolar non-ketotic diabetic coma (HONK). Although they are usually described as separate entities, there is considerable overlap in their pathogenesis and treatment. For example, although "hyperosmolarity" is only specified in HONK, it is also an important feature of DKA and, in both conditions, results from progressive hyperglycaemic dehydration. Similarly, a major component of the treatment of both is fluid and electrolyte replacement. Differences arise from the time over which the metabolic disturbance develops—hours or days in DKA, days or weeks in HONK—and the type of patient who is typically affected. For clarity, DKA and HONK will be described separately.

Diabetic ketoacidosis

Incidence and prevalence

Some general points can be drawn from a large population-based survey in Rhode Island, USA, an area with a well-defined population, in which all cases of DKA were identified in one year.[1] This survey found that DKA:

- accounted for 152 of 9663 (1.6%) diabetic admissions
- had an annual incidence of 46 per 10 000 diabetics
- had a female predominance of 2:1
- was the presenting feature of diabetes in 20% of cases
- was a recurrent problem in 15% of patients
- occurred most commonly in patients <15 years old.

Most surveys have found a striking increase in admission for uncontrolled diabetes in adolescence. For example, a community-based study in Rochester, Minnesota, found an incidence of DKA of 13.4/1000/year in those diagnosed <30 years of age and 3.3/1000/year in those diagnosed >30 years.[2]

Mortality

In the pre-insulin era type 1 diabetes was uniformly fatal, and the commonest cause of death was ketoacidotic coma. Following the introduction of insulin in 1922 and increased understanding of the pathogenesis of DKA, mortality fell rapidly to around 30% by 1932 and to 10% by the late 1970s.

Ketoacidosis remains a significant cause of death in diabetes especially in those >50 years of age, where mortality rates approach 20%. Much of this excess mortality results from co-incident or precipitating disease (e.g. myocardial infarction).

A 1981 survey of deaths of type 1 diabetes patients <50 years of age in the UK found that 15% were due to DKA.[3] In patients aged <20, DKA accounted for 16 of 23 deaths. Clinical errors in fluid administration, inadequate potassium replacement leading to hypokalaemic cardiac arrest, delay in insulin administration and aspiration pneumonia were contributory factors in 40% of cases. Poor documentation was a feature of fatal cases suggesting inadequate medical care.

Pathophysiology

DKA results from the combined effects of insulin deficiency and increased counterregulatory hormones (Figure 3.1). The clinical picture can be worked out logically if you look at the biochemistry.

Insulin deficiency
The effects of insulin deficiency are easily seen in studies of insulin withdrawal in patients with type 1 diabetes. Within one hour of intravenous insulin withdrawal, blood glucose concentrations increase as a result of:

- increased hepatic glucose production from glycogen (glycogenolysis)
- increased hepatic glucose synthesis from amino acids (gluconeogenesis)
- reduced uptake of glucose into skeletal muscle and fat.

47

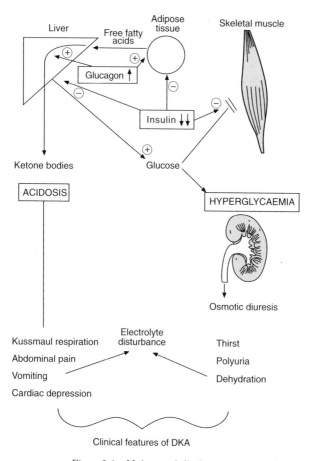

Figure 3.1   Major metabolic derangements causing DKA.

The resulting hyperglycaemia leads to an increased urine output owing to an osmotic diuresis which initially acts as a "safety valve". Increased losses of fluid in the urine stimulate thirst which can help to maintain hydration as long as the patient is not vomiting. The critical factor is the onset of vomiting, often related to worsening acidosis, which causes more rapid dehydration, prerenal failure and further rise in blood glucose.

Excess counterregulatory hormones

Glucagon concentrations are invariably raised and contribute to the speed of onset and severity of DKA. In the presence of severe insulin deficiency, glucagon stimulates hepatic gluconeogenesis and worsens hyperglycaemia. Glucagon is also lipolytic and stimulates release of free fatty acids into the circulation, where they are used as a substrate for ketone body synthesis in the liver. There are three ketone bodies, all of which are organic acids:

- acetoacetone
- beta-hydroxybutyrate
- acetone.

Ketone body concentrations increase within one to two hours of insulin withdrawal, and are the principal cause of metabolic acidosis. Usually all three are increased but occasionally beta-hydroxbutyrate concentrations are disproportionately elevated. This may create a diagnostic problem, since the nitroprusside reaction for ketones does not react with beta-hydroxybutyrate. In these circumstances, clinical evaluation and laboratory assessment are needed to exclude other causes of a metabolic acidosis (e.g. measurement of renal function, lactate and salicylate concentrations).

The significance of glucagon in the pathogenesis of DKA has been studied in patients who have diabetes as a result of a total pancreatectomy. Such patients can still develop DKA but, because of the absolute lack of pancreatic glucagon, the rate of onset is much slower than is seen in patients with classical type 1 diabetes (Figure 3.2).

Fluid and electrolyte loss

Patients with DKA are always dehydrated mainly because of the osmotic diuresis. Vomiting may worsen fluid and electroyte loss in some patients. Table 3.1 shows typical losses of fluid and electrolytes in DKA.

Precipitating factors

Most surveys find similar underlying reasons for the development of DKA but the relative proportions vary according to the age of the population studied, and the criteria for diagnosing intercurrent illness. A list of common precipitants is shown in Table 3.2.

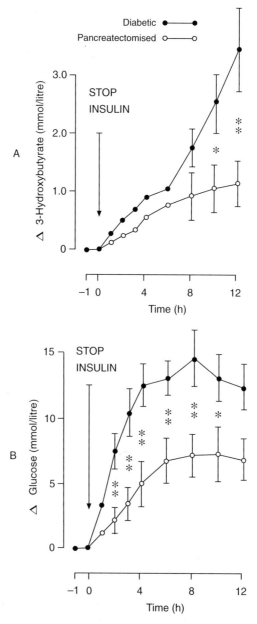

Figure 3.2   Changes (Δ) in blood concentrations (mean ± SEM) of 3-hydroxybutyrate (A) and glucose (B) in six patients with juvenile-type diabetes and four pancreatectomised patients after insulin withdrawal. (*P<0.05; **P<0.02).

Table 3.1   Losses of fluid and electrolytes in DKA

Fluid/electrolytes	Estimated deficit
Total body water	5–7 litres
Sodium	700–1000 mmol/litre
Potassium	250–500 mmol/litre
Chloride	500–700 mmol/litre
Calcium	50–150 mmol/litre
Phosphate	50–150 mmol/litre

Table 3.2   Causes of DKA in 746 episodes in Birmingham, UK, between 1971 and 1985[4]

Cause	Percentage (%)
Infection	28
Errors in management by patient or medical advisor	13
Myocardial infarction	1
Newly diagnosed type 1 diabetes	10
Miscellaneous	5
No cause found	43

Intercurrent illness causes hyperglycaemia and a deterioration of diabetic control which usually requires patients to increase their insulin dose, even if they are off their food or vomiting. All patients with type 1 diabetes need to be aware of their "sick-day rules" (see p. 69), the most important one being: **Never stop your insulin**. However, some patients are reluctant to inject if they are not eating and, sometimes, doctors, nurses or friends (incorrectly) offer this advice.

How far intercurrent illness is responsible for precipitating DKA depends on the diagnostic precision used to define the illness. As detailed below, a raised white count is common in pure DKA and does not necessarily indicate infection. Objective evidence of intercurrent illness is uncommon in patients <25 years of age, in whom new presentation or the mistaken or deliberate omission of insulin are the commonest precipitants. With increasing age, intercurrent illness, often associated with infection or myocardial infarction, assumes more importance as a precipitant, and may account for up to 50% of DKA admissions.

51

Some of the "no cause found" cases are due to deliberate omission or reduction of insulin to get away from stress at home or as part of an eating disorder. Such manipulation and the resulting admission with DKA are a powerful means of escaping a difficult social situation or of seeking attention, and are most commonly seen in adolescent girls with type 1 diabetes. Reading the medical notes may reveal previous admissions with DKA, and small numbers of such patients can significantly increase annual admissions of DKA in a diabetes unit. A few patients have long-term poor glycaemic control and will often have urinary ketones in "routine" outpatient samples. Some have a primary eating disorder (anorexia or bulimia nervosa) which they are likely to conceal and, as a result of erratic diet and insulin therapy, they are often "on the edge" of ketoacidosis.

Continuous subcutaneous insulin infusion therapy (CSII) which is sometimes used in Europe and the USA presents particular risks with respect to DKA. Unlike patients using insulin injections, those using CSII have no depot of insulin in subcutaneous tissues. In the event of pump failure or intercurrent illness, DKA may develop rapidly over a few hours.[5] Not surprisingly, patients who have recently transferred to CSII and are "on the learning curve" are at greatest risk, and the same applies to centres which offer the service.

Diagnosis

A concise history and rapid clinical assessment are essential. In a "typical" presentation, the diagnosis is usually straightforward. There is usually a short period of 12–24 hours when the symptoms of hyperglycaemia develop, followed by the onset of vomiting and acidotic breathing.

Clinical features of DKA include:

- polyuria, thirst, nocturia
- blurring of vision
- cramps in legs
- shortness of breath
- nausea and vomiting
- abdominal pain.

Specific problems with presentation

The previously undiagnosed

Such patients may account for up to 15% of admissions with DKA. The average GP will encounter a new case of type 1 diabetes every 20 years, and a high index of suspicion is needed. Often the diagnosis is delayed because simple tests for glycosuria and ketonuria are not performed. The following case illustrates the point.

Case Study 7

A 16-year-old adolescent complained of a one-week history of tiredness and thirst. He was reviewed by his GP who diagnosed a viral infection and advised rest. Over the next few days his condition deteriorated and a second doctor was asked to visit. The youth had developed mild abdominal pain and had vomited once. The second physician tested the urine for protein (but not glucose), found none and recommended no change in treatment. Over the next two days the vomiting and abdominal pain worsened; he became drowsy and was taken to casualty, where severe DKA was diagnosed.

Children

DKA can develop within a few hours and precipitants, such as otitis media or tonsillitis, should be sought. Treatment principles are similar to that in adults with adjustment of fluid replacement needs according to the child's age and body weight. Such patients are usually managed best on a paediatric intensive care unit.

Pregnancy

The development of DKA during pregnancy in women with type 1 diabetes is associated with a fetal mortality of >50%. Comprehensive education about managing intercurrent illness needs to be provided before or during pregnancy: the mother needs to know how to test for ketones, and open access should be available to medical or obstetric units at all times. The principles of treatment are the same as those in non-pregnant women.[6]

The elderly

Symptoms of DKA in the elderly can be less obvious than in the younger population. For example, thirst is often less marked, whilst urinary frequency can often be put down to prostatism in men or infection in women. Symptoms may be misinterpreted so that for example, acidotic breathing may be thought to be due to heart failure or a chest infection, whilst drowsiness or confusion may be misdiagnosed as cerebrovascular disease.

The elderly who develop DKA are also more likely than younger people to have an intercurrent illness, and it is important to remember that infection may precipitate DKA in those with type 2 diabetes. To avoid such diagnostic problems, the urine should *always* be tested for ketones in anybody with diabetes who is unwell, although this may present obvious practical difficulties for a GP visiting an elderly ill person at home.

Unrecognised severity

The clinical severity of DKA depends more on the degree of acidosis than the blood glucose. If too much emphasis is placed on the blood glucose concentration, patients (and their physicians) may be falsely reassured as is illustrated in the following case.

Case Study 8

A 28-year-old woman with known diabetes called her GP because of thirst, abdominal pain and breathlessness. She had had influenza-type symptoms for the previous two days; she had been monitoring her blood glucose but had not tested her urine for ketones. The GP performed a capillary blood glucose measurement and was reassured to find that it was only 17 mmol/litre. The following day her condition worsened and she was admitted as an emergency in a semiconscious state with an arterial pH of 6.8 and a blood glucose of 15.4 mmol/litre.

The clear message is that **patients with uncontrolled diabetes need to be assessed for both hyperglycaemia and the severity of the metabolic acidosis**.

Abdominal pain

This is relatively common as a symptom of DKA and may cause diagnostic difficulties. The pain is usually generalised or epigastric, and may be associated with vomiting. On occasion the abdomen may be rigid and the bowel sounds infrequent or absent. The dilemma is whether the pain is related solely to DKA or whether an intra-abdominal "event" may be responsible for the pain (and indirectly the DKA). Diagnostic difficulty can increase when a markedly raised amylase is found on initial blood tests, suggesting the possibility of pancreatitis (see below).

Effective treatment of DKA should lessen or cure the abdominal pain within 6–12 hours. If it persists or worsens after this time, a surgical condition is more likely, but the delay is beneficial since it allows for proper rehydration and better blood glucose control prior to emergency surgery.

Level of consciousness

Many patients with DKA are drowsy and occasionally confused at presentation but true "coma" is uncommon, affecting <10%. Whether DKA leads to an altered level of consciousness depends on the severity of the underlying metabolic disturbance. The most reliable predictor is the plasma osmolality which can be readily calculated from the patient's glucose, urea and electrolyte concentrations (in millimoles/litre) using the equation:

$$\text{Osmolality} = 2(Na + K) + urea + glucose$$

Calculated or measured osmolalities >340 mosm/litre are likely to be associated with altered levels of consciousness.

Clinical assessment (Box 3.1)

Patients with suspected DKA should be assessed quickly to confirm the diagnosis so that treatment can be started as soon as possible. A brief history should be taken followed by a clinical examination looking for obvious precipitating illness. The typical patient is drowsy, flushed and dehydrated with Kussmaul

---

Box 3.1 Clinical features indicating severe DKA

- Tachycardia
- Small volume pulse
- Postural or supine hypotension
- Cool peripheries
- Peripheral cyanosis
- Kussmaul respiration
- Drowsiness

respiration. The ability to smell acetone on the breath is idiosyncratic and should not be relied upon as a substitute for measuring urine or plasma ketones.

Dehydration is always present and measurement of pulse and blood pressure are essential to assess the extent of fluid loss. If possible, both supine and erect blood pressures should be recorded. Other features suggesting severe dehydration include cold extremities, peripheral cyanosis, a thready pulse and oliguria.

Investigations

Essential

- **Glucose:** To support the diagnosis of DKA and provide a baseline to assess response to treatment. Ward-based reflectance meters can underestimate the blood glucose in the presence of DKA and a sample must be sent to the laboratory.
- **Electrolytes:** Despite large urinary losses of sodium, plasma concentrations are usually normal or slightly low, ranging from 130 to 140 mmol/litre. Hyperglycaemia also contributes to the development of hyponatraemia, because the osmotic gradient moves water from the intracellular compartment and dilutes extracellular solutes. As a rule of thumb, 1.5 mmol/litre should be subtracted from the measured sodium concentration for every 5.0 mmol/litre of glucose over 5.5 mmol/litre in the patient's sample.

  Plasma potassium is usually at the upper end of normal or slightly increased (Table 3.3). It is important to emphasise that the plasma potassium does **not** reflect the total body potassium deficit which is **always** present. However, patients with hypokalaemia at presentation are always severely potassium deficient and require energetic replacement therapy during treatment.

Table 3.3   Percentage of patients with DKA who have disturbances of plasma potassium at presentation[7]

Plasma potassium	Percentage (%)
Hypokalaemia	5–10
Normal potassium	70–80
Hyperkalaemia	10–20

- **Plasma urea:** Usually raised as a feature of prerenal impairment secondary to dehydration.
- **Venous bicarbonate:** To assess the severity of the acidosis. In many studies a value of $\leqslant 15$ mmol/litre is accepted to define DKA.
- **Urinary and plasma ketones:** Best measured with a nitroprusside-based reaction such as Ketostix.
- **Blood cultures:** To identify possible underlying infection which may have precipitated DKA. Diagnosis of infection in DKA is difficult, since fever may not appear until after rehydration, and the white cell count is usually raised in the absence of infection.

Optional depending on clinical circumstance

- **Arterial blood gases:** Should be reserved for semiconscious patients or cases where there is no clinical improvement despite fluid and electrolyte replacement plus insulin after two to three hours.
- **Urine microscopy and culture:** Not necessary if the urine is clear on gross inspection, but may be needed to confirm urinary tract infection in selected cases.
- **ECG:** To exclude underlying silent myocardial infarction, especially in those >40 years of age or with long duration of diabetes.
- **Chest X-ray:** If there are signs of infection.

Potentially misleading

- **White cell count:** Often raised to 15–20 000 with a neutrophil leucocytosis. Does not signify infection in the absence of obvious clinical signs.
- **Amylase:** May be raised two- to three-fold, and is mainly of salivary gland origin. In a patient with abdominal pain from DKA, this may cause diagnostic confusion (see comments pp. 54–55).
- **Creatinine:** There is a potential risk of interference by raised plasma ketones, although modern methods have largely overcome this problem. If in doubt check with your local laboratory.
- **Lipids:** Usually deranged in uncontrolled diabetes. Triglyceride concentrations are usually raised but cholesterol remains normal. Occasionally, triglycerides may be grossly elevated (>50 mmol/litre), and the serum has a milky appearance

from the accumulation of VLDL and chylomicrons (diabetic lipaemia). The major complication of diabetic lipaemia is pancreatitis, but the condition may also be associated with hepatosplenomegaly, eruptive xanthomata and memory impairment. The lipid abnormalities respond rapidly to insulin therapy.

Treatment

Treatment of DKA is based on replacement of fluid, electrolytes and insulin to treat the dehydration, hyperglycaemia and acid-base disturbance. Before discussing these in detail several general points should be made:

- Patients with "mild or moderate" DKA, who are conscious, able to give an account of their illness and whose blood chemistry is not markedly deranged, can be treated on a general medical ward. Those with severe DKA, who are semiconscious, with marked hypotension, and severe acidosis or electrolyte disturbance (particularly hypokalaemia), should be treated on a High Dependency Unit with ECG monitoring and staff trained to interpret the trace.
- Treatment should correct the metabolic disturbance over 12–24 hours, depending on the severity of the episode.
- During the first 24 hours all patients with DKA need close supervision by doctors and nurses and regular monitoring of their electrolytes and glucose concentrations.
- Guidelines can help to select appropriate treatment options *but are no substitute for clinical judgement* depending on the condition of the individual patient.

Fluids

The free water deficit in DKA averages 5–7 litres. Rehydration is the first priority and helps to lower blood glucose by dilution and improving glomerular filtration, thereby encouraging glucose loss in the urine. Most of the fall of blood glucose in the first one to two hours of treatment is due to dilution.

Which fluid is best? In most cases isotonic saline should be used (Table 3.4). Where severe hypotension is present on admission (systolic BP <80 mmHg), rapid infusion rates should be used to

58

Table 3.4 Suggested fluid replacement during the first 24 hours

	Infusion fluid	Volume (ml)	Additives (mmol/KCl)	To be infused over
1	0.9% saline	500	Nil	10 min
2	0.9% saline	1000	20–40	1–2 h
3	0.9% saline	1000	20–40	1–2 h
4	0.9% saline	1000	20–40	2–4 h
5	0.9% saline	1000	20–40	2–4 h
6	0.9% saline	1000	20–40	2–4 h
			or	
	5% dextrose	1000	20–40	4–6 h

restore renal blood flow, and occasionally infusion of a plasma expander (for example 500 ml Haemaccel) may be necessary until blood pressure increases to >100 mmHg. Isotonic saline should then be substituted.

Occasionally during treatment hypernatraemia develops as a result of free water moving to the extravascular and intracellular compartments. If plasma sodium rises to >150 mmol/litre, 0.45% saline should be used instead of isotonic saline.

When blood glucose falls to 15 mmol/litre, the infusion fluid should be changed to 5% dextrose. The blood glucose should be maintained in the range 10–15 mmol/litre until full recovery has been achieved, in order to lessen the risk of cerebral oedema (see p. 64).

Potassium

Irrespective of the plasma concentration, total body potassium is **always** markedly depleted, with a deficit ranging from 3 to 12 mmol/kg. Potassium loss occurs primarily because of the osmotic diuresis but plasma concentrations are also affected by other factors relating to the acidotic state (Table 3.5).

Since potassium is predominantly an intracellular ion, the severity of total body potassium loss is not represented in the serum potassium concentration, which is usually at the upper end of the normal range at presentation. Approximately 2% of patients with DKA will have significant hyperkalaemia (K>6.0 mmol/litre,) often as a result of severe dehydration and prerenal impairment.

Hypokalaemia has been reported in about 5% of cases of DKA and is a potential danger since, with rehydration and insulin, serum

Table 3.5   Factors which influence plasma potassium concentrations in DKA

Cause	Mechanism	Consequence
Insulin deficiency	Prevents potassium entry into cells	Loss of K+ from cells
Metabolic acidosis	Exchange of hydrogen for potassium ions	Loss of K+ from cells
Osmotic diuresis	Major route of potassium losses	Urinary K+ loss
Vomiting	Acidosis	Gastric K+ loss
Renal impairment	Dehydration	Reduced renal K+ loss

potassium concentrations fall further, putting the patient at risk of hypokalaemic cardiac arrest.

Potassium replacement during early treatment of DKA is **vital**. Early replacement should be prescribed once the patient's serum potassium is known, and should begin with the second and subsequent bags of fluid. A suggested regimen for potassium replacement is shown in Table 3.6, but it must be emphasised that regular laboratory monitoring (every four to six hours during the first 12 hours) is essential to avoid serious hypokalaemia during treatment.

Table 3.6   Suggested regimen for potassium replacement

Plasma potassium (mmol/litre)	Replacement needed (mmol/litre intravenous fluid)
>5.5	None
3.5–5.5	20
<3.5	40

Oral potassium supplements (2–4 g/day) should be given for seven days after an episode of severe DKA to fully replenish total body potassium.

Insulin

Insulin is an essential part of treatment of DKA, since it will help to lower blood glucose and, importantly, it will inhibit ketogenesis and begin to reverse the effects of the metabolic acidosis. Modern approaches are based on low dose insulin regimens[8] which can be given by continuous intravenous infusion or, where resources are limited, by hourly intramuscular injection. Such regimens are associated with much less risk of inducing severe hypokalaemia and hypoglycaemia compared with regimens used until the 1970s when doses of 50–100 units/h of insulin were given.

On arrival in the emergency room, patients with a confirmed diagnosis of DKA should be given a loading dose of 10 units soluble insulin intramuscularly. Subcutaneous injections in patients with dehydration are absorbed slowly and erratically and should be avoided. Further insulin should ideally be given intravenously and, where facilities for infusion by a syringe driver are available, a convenient regimen is to dilute 50 units of insulin to a volume of 50 ml in isotonic saline. This can be infused so the number of ml/h equates to the number of units of insulin/h (Table 3.7).

Table 3.7   Sliding scale for insulin administration

Blood glucose (mmol/litre)	Insulin infusion rate (units/h)
0–3.9	0.5
4.0–6.9	1.0
7.0–9.9	2.0
10.0–14.9	3.0
15.0–19.9	4.0
>20.0	5.0

The infusion rate should be adjusted until laboratory blood glucose results fall into the range when capillary blood glucose can be measured with a reflectance meter. Once blood glucose falls to 15 mmol/litre, the infusion fluid should be changed to 5% glucose, and the insulin infusion adjusted to maintain the blood glucose in the range of 10–15 mmol/litre.

One disadvantage of a conventional intravenous insulin sliding scale is that the patient receives less insulin as the blood glucose decreases, particularly when the initial glucose is not very high but there is a severe metabolic acidosis; the reduced insulin infusion rates may delay recovery of the acidosis. In this situation it can be helpful to "clamp" the insulin infusion rate at, for example 5 units/h to suppress lipolysis. Hypoglycaemia can be prevented by infusing sufficient glucose as a 5 or 10% solution (250–500 ml/h) until the arterial pH has risen to >7.2.

In all patients the insulin infusion should be continued until they are eating and drinking. Subcutaneous insulin can be started at this stage. Note that when an intravenous infusion is stopped the patient becomes totally insulin deficient within 10 minutes. To prevent this the insulin infusion should be continued for one to two hours after the first subcutaneous injection. Insulin resistance is present in most cases of DKA because of the effects of counterregulatory hormones and acidosis.[9] It is not usually clinically important during acute management, but needs to be taken into account when an intravenous is being swapped to a subcutaneous regimen; a 10% increase in usual insulin doses is often needed for several days after an episode of DKA.

Where facilities for intravenous insulin are unavailable, the above regimen can be adapted by using hourly intramuscular injections of soluble insulin (10 units) until blood glucose falls to the desired range of 10–15 mmol/litre.

Bicarbonate

The role of sodium bicarbonate in treating acidosis in DKA has been controversial for over 50 years.[10] Several trials have failed to show clinical benefit from administration of bicarbonate, and there are theoretical reasons why it may be counterproductive:

- When extracellular acidosis is corrected, bicarbonate causes increased potassium uptake by cells and may worsen hypokalaemia, especially when given with intravenous rehydration and insulin.
- There may be a paradoxical worsening of CSF acidosis because of the differential permeability of the blood–brain barrier to CO_2.
- Acidosis causes a shift in the oxygen dissociation curve for haemoglobin; this is compensated for by a decrease in red cell 2,3-diphosphoglycerate (2,3-DPG). Rapid correction of acidosis with bicarbonate will shift the dissociation curve to the left and, since 2,3-DPG levels take several days to correct, tissue oxygen delivery may be reduced.

On the other hand, severe acidosis depresses cardiac function and can cause prolonged hypotension despite adequate fluid replacement. For this reason, many authorities suggest that bicarbonate be reserved for cases with severe acidosis (pH<6.9) that have not responded to rehydration and insulin, but this recommendation is not evidence based. A suggested approach to severe acidosis is as follows:

- Measure arterial pH in patients who remain hypotensive despite fluid replacement.
- Ensure adequate insulin administration. An intravenous insulin infusion rate of 5 units/h, with concurrent administration of 10%

dextrose to maintain blood glucose concentrations if necessary, should be used.

- If hypotension persists, give 500 ml *isotonic* (1.4%) sodium bicarbonate and assess the response of arterial pH and cardio-vascular function. Ensure adequate K+ replacement is given to avoid severe hypokalaemia and cardiac arrhythmias.
- Do not use *hypertonic* (8.4%) sodium bicarbonate because it causes thrombosis of the peripheral veins, and the excessive sodium load may precipitate pulmonary oedema in vulnerable patients.
- Administration of bicarbonate should ideally be supervised in a high dependency or intensive care unit where invasive cardiac monitoring is possible.

General measures

A number of additional measures need to be considered in some patients with DKA, usually those with more severe metabolic disturbance.

- **Nasogastric tube:** Should be considered in patients who are drowsy and have been vomiting. Acute gastric dilatation is common in DKA with the associated risk of aspiration of gastric contents. A succussion splash may be elicited in the abdomen.
- **Urinary catheter:** Is usually unnecessary but should be considered in the elderly, in those with impaired renal function or prolonged hypotension unresponsive to fluid challenge.
- **Invasive cardiac monitoring:** Internal jugular or Swan-Ganz catheters for monitoring are occasionally needed to guide fluid replacement, particularly in patients with severe acute or chronic cardiac failure, renal failure or septic shock, and in those who remain hypotensive despite adequate fluid replacement as a result of severe acidosis.
- **Low dose heparin:** Should be given to patients at risk of venous thrombosis, because DKA is often associated with low grade disseminated intravascular coagulation. Patients at particular risk include the elderly, those with a past history of thromboembolic disease, and those with severe dehydration or immobility.

Finally and self-evidently, if an underlying organic cause for DKA is identified, appropriate therapy is required.

Monitoring of treatment

It cannot be emphasised too strongly that the key to successful treatment of DKA is careful monitoring and regular assessment by an enthusiastic physician. In the first 12 hours, laboratory measurement of glucose, electrolytes and renal function is needed with particular emphasis on potassium. Also, whilst rehydration is in progress, the patient should be regularly assessed: look for signs of adequate (blood pressure, urine output) or excessive fluid replacement (raised venous pressure, basal crackles). A suggested monitoring schedule is shown in Table 3.8, but this needs to be tailored to individual patients. For example, a patient with hypo- or hyperkalaemia would require potassium checks every two hours for the first few hours of therapy, to ensure adequate and safe replacement.

Table 3.8   Monitoring schedule for patient's treatment

Hours	Glucose	U + E	Venous bicarbonate	Urine ketones	Clinical assessment
0	+	+	+	+	+
1	+				
2	+	+			+
3	+				
4	+	+	+	+	+
6	+				
8	+	+	+	+	+
16	+	+		+	+
24	+	+	+	+	+

Abbreviations: U + E: Urea & electrolytes

A serial data sheet (Figure 3.3), on which the treatment regimen together with the results of laboratory tests and clinical observations can be monitored, greatly assists effective monitoring of patients with DKA.

Complications

A number of complications may arise from DKA or its treatment.

Cerebral oedema

This usually affects young patients, especially children. Clinically significant cerebral oedema occurs in about 1% admissions for DKA in children, in whom it is associated with a mortality

Sliding Scale Insulin Prescription Card

This sliding scale will be administered intravenously unless specified on this chart.

Enter the sliding scale in the first two columns. If anything needs to be altered, cross out all of that scale then rewrite it. If no insulin is to be given at a certain level, write 'NIL' – do not leave blank.

Blood glucose	Insulin rate (units/h)	Blood glucose	Insulin rate (ml/h)	Blood glucose	Insulin rate (units/h)
Check glucose every:	h		h		h
Date					
Signature					

Insulin infusions are continuous and made up of **50 units soluble insulin (Actrapid) in 50 ml of 0.9% saline.** The signature below authorises that this insulin infusion prescription is to be repeated until the sliding scale is stopped by a doctor.

Doctor's signature: [   ]

Insulin infusion record

This record must be kept by the **nursing staff**. When it is full, start a new insulin card and attach it to this one.

Insulin batch no.	Saline batch no.	Time infusion started	Date	Signed

Advice to prescriber

Suggested **DKA** insulin regime

BM	Rate (units/h)
0–3.9	0.5
4–8	1
8.1–12	2
12.1–16	3
16.1+	4

Remember that in **hyperosmolar non-ketosis (HONK)** patients are usually very sensitive to i.v. insulin: 0.5–1 unit/h may be sufficient to lower blood glucose by 5 mmol/h.

For further advice, consult the *Junior Physician's Handbook* or someone more experienced.

Now complete the fluid prescription and data record within this prescription card

Figure 3.3   Example of a combined fluid and insulin prescription chart and laboratory data sheet for the treatment and monitoring of patients with DKA.

Data Record

When you have checked or changed the insulin infusion rate, initial the box.

Today's Date:

Time	Insulin infusion			Results								Intake (ml)			Output (ml)			
	Rate (units/h)	BM strip	Signed	Lab Glucose	Na	K	Urea	Creat	Bicarb	Urine ketones		i.v. fluid	Oral fluid	Running total	Urine vol.	Other	Running total	
												24 h total			24 h total			

Figure 3.3 continued

66

approaching 90%.[11] The aetiology is disputed but it has been linked to rapid infusion of hypotonic fluid causing a rapid fall in plasma osmolality, which leads to enhanced uptake of water in the brain.[12] Cerebral oedema is rare, if blood glucose is maintained at about 15 mmol/litre for the first 48 hours. In practice this can be achieved if infusion fluid is changed from isotonic saline to 5% glucose, once the plasma glucose has fallen to 15 mmol/litre.

Symptoms typically develop during the first 12 hours of treatment and usually present as a deterioration in consciousness in a child or adolescent who initially seemed to be responding well. Cerebral imaging with CT or MRI scanning is mandatory to confirm oedema and exclude other causes of loss of consciousness. Treatment of established cerebral oedema should include:

- reducing the intravenous fluid infusion rate;
- using intravenous infusions of mannitol;
- dexamethasone (which requires increases in insulin doses), and
- ventilatory support to maintain hypocapnia.

Intracerebral pressure monitoring may guide treatment if this is available.

Adult respiratory distress syndrome

The typical presentation includes rapidly progressive shortness of breath, worsening hypoxia and bilateral alveolar pulmonary shadowing. The pathophysiology is unclear but may be related to falling colloid osmotic pressure and rising left atrial pressure from excessively rapid fluid replacement. An associated alveolar–capillary perfusion defect from severe acidosis has also been implicated. Treatment involves ventilatory support with positive end expiratory pressures, together with high inspired oxygen concentrations. Central pressure monitoring, if available, is essential in monitoring fluid balance but, even with full intensive care support, mortality is high.

Gastric stasis

Acute abdominal distension, copious vomiting, and a high risk of aspiration pneumonia with a succussion splash evident on abdominal examination are typical. Treatment is to pass a nasogastric tube and aspirate stomach contents, and this should be done in any patient who is excessively drowsy or unconscious.

Non-traumatic rhabdomyolysis

The diagnosis of this rare complication is based on a raised creatine kinase, in the absence of a history or ECG evidence of acute myocardial infarction. Rarely, the associated myoglobinaemia (together with dehydration) may cause acute renal failure.

Mediastinal surgical emphysema

Approximately 30 cases of spontaneous surgical emphysema have been described. It usually occurs in patients with severe acidosis, prolonged hyperventilation and vomiting. Increased alveolar pressure, with damage to alveolar walls and escape of air into interstitial lung tissue, has been suggested as a possible mechanism. The chest and neck are usually affected and a chest X-ray may also reveal mediastinal emphysema. Chest pain is reported in about 30% of cases and usually develops 24–48 hours after effective treatment of DKA. A typical pericardial crunching noise (Hamman's sign) may be heard over the apex where mediastinal emphysema is present. Spontaneous resolution occurs over 7–10 days and no specific therapy is needed.

Education/prevention

Prevention is better than cure and, once the metabolic disturbance has been treated, it is important to clarify events leading up to the admission to determine the cause of the DKA and the need for (re-)education. Was the admission precipitated by an intercurrent illness, a failure of education or self-inflicted by omission of insulin, or for another reason? For known type 1 diabetes patients, it is a good opportunity to reinforce "sick day rules", and ideally written information should be provided (Box 3.2). Revision of these simple guidelines during subsequent consultations is also important.

Routine urine testing for ketones is unnecessary, but all patients with type 1 diabetes should understand the significance of ketones, and be taught urine testing with Ketostix so they can test during intercurrent illness. Persistent ketonuria should prompt a medical opinion.

Box 3.2 Sick day rules

Never stop your insulin

- Measure blood glucose at least four times each day (pre-breakfast, lunch, tea and bed).
- Depending on the result, take the following action:
  - Blood glucose <11 mmol/litre—give normal insulin
  - Blood glucose between 11 and 17 mmol/litre—4 units *extra* of clear insulin
  - Blood glucose >17 mmol/litre—6 units *extra* of clear insulin
- If you don't feel like eating, replace your normal meals with fluids, such as milk, lucozade, fruit juice which should be taken every one or two hours. Also drink plenty of sugar free liquids.
- If you have a temperature, take two paracetamol up to four times each day.
- If your bloods are continuously more than 17 mmol/litre, or you are being sick, or you are unsure of what to do, contact your diabetes nurse specialist or general practitioner

Hyperosmolar non-ketotic diabetic coma

Hyperosmolar non-ketotic (HONK) diabetic coma is the second major clinical presentation of uncontrolled diabetes.

Incidence and prevalence

HONK is less common than DKA and almost exclusively seen in patients >60 years of age. There is a slight female preponderance probably due to the increased life-expectancy of women compared with men, and, in about 30%, it is the initial presentation of type 2 diabetes. A number of precipitating factors have been linked to the development of HONK (Table 3.9).

Elderly patients are also at increased risk of developing HONK because of impaired perception of thirst, resulting in progressive dehydration in the face of a persistent osmotic diuresis.

Pathophysiology

The essential clinical features of HONK are described in its acronym. As mentioned in the introduction, there are similarities between HONK and DKA including hyperglycaemia, dehydration

Table 3.9 Precipitating factors in HONK

Precipitating event	Mechanism
Drugs	
Beta-blockers	Reduce insulin secretion
Thiazide or loop diuretics	Reduce insulin secretion
Corticosteroids	Increase insulin resistance
Enteral or parenteral feeding	Increases osmotic load
Excessive intravenous glucose administration	Increases osmotic load
Post-cardiac surgery	Administration of dextrose containing fluids
Being in a nursing home	

and electrolyte losses, and many principles of treatment are similar. The conditions do differ in a number of important respects (Table 3.10).

As with DKA, an osmotic diuresis is central to the pathogenesis but this develops more slowly. It is not unusual to elicit a history of progressive worsening health and increasing confusion over two or three weeks. Dehydration may be made worse by limited access to water and by the reduced perception of thirst in the elderly. Some patients who do try to quench their thirst "fan the flames" of progressive hyperglycaemia by choosing high glucose-containing drinks.

HONK is characterised by marked hyperglycaemia and loss of water of up to 25% of body weight in severe cases. Water is lost from the intravascular compartment via the kidney by osmotic diuresis, but the osmotic gradient draws water from both intracellular and extracellular sites, leading to profound dehydration, which ultimately causes hypotension and prerenal failure. This further increases the hyperglycaemia by reducing renal

Table 3.10 Differences between DKA and HONK

Factors	DKA	HONK
Age	Any age	Usually >60 years
Presentation	Hours or days	Days or weeks
Mortality	5% overall	50%
Glucose	High	Very high
Osmolality	High	Very high
Serum sodium	Normal or low	Normal or high
Bicarbonate	<15	Normal or slightly low
Ketonuria	+ + + +	None or +
Treatment	Insulin	Diet $\pm$ oral hypoglycaemics

Table 3.11 Possible mechanisms for failure of ketone body formation in HONK

Reason	Mechanism
Higher portal insulin concentrations	Reduced hepatic ketogenesis
Lower counterregulatory hormones	Less lipid breakdown and reduced stimulation of hepatic ketogenesis
High osmolality suppressing lipolysis	Less free fatty acid substrate for hepatic ketogenesis

glucose clearance. A key difference in HONK is the lack of significant ketone body production compared to that in DKA. Several mechanisms have been suggested to account for this (Table 3.11).

Problems with presentation

In as many as 40% of cases, a clinical presentation with HONK may be the first evidence of diabetes. In a confused elderly patient, obtaining a clear history of typical diabetic symptoms can be difficult, and a high index of suspicion is needed. HONK should form part of the differential diagnosis of a wide range of neurological presentations in the elderly. Confusion and disorientation are common and, as with DKA, the plasma osmolality most closely determines the presence or absence of a reduced level of consciousness. Coma is associated with plasma osmolalities >340 mosm/kg.

A number of focal neurological findings have been reported with HONK, as the following case report shows.

Case Study 9

A 54-year-old Afro-Caribbean taxi driver was found slumped over the steering wheel of his car. The emergency services were called but, during his transfer to hospital, he had two self-limiting grand mal seizures. On arrival in casualty he was drowsy and unresponsive to commands. No clear history was available. He was hypotensive and clinically dehydrated. Urgent biochemistry revealed a blood glucose of 98.5 mmol/litre, with biochemical features of prerenal renal failure. He was transferred to a high dependency unit where he was rehydrated and a low-dose insulin infusion was started. He made a full recovery.

It emerged that he had been feeling unwell, thirsty and tired for several weeks. He had been quenching his thirst with "off-the-shelf" lemonade. There was no history of previous seizures or other neurological illness.

71

In addition to focal seizures, other neurological abnormalities, including aphasia, hemiparesis, homonomous hemianopia, nystagmus and extensor Babinski responses, have been described in HONK.[13] The cause of these focal neurological symptoms is unknown but complete resolution is usual. Laboratory measurement of blood glucose is an essential investigation in any elderly patient with altered CNS function.

Finally it is important to emphasise that laboratory blood glucose measurements are needed rather than a capillary blood glucose measurement. The gross elevations of blood glucose, often >50 mmol/litre in HONK, can result in underestimation if test strips read by a reflectance meter are relied on as the sole measure for blood glucose.

Investigations

These are similar to those outlined in the investigation of DKA. A number of points should be made:

- **Glucose:** There is some overlap but glucose concentrations are often higher than those seen in DKA and are often >50 mmol/litre. The author has seen a glucose concentration of 102 mmol/litre (from which the patient made a good recovery).
- **Sodium:** Unlike in DKA, sodium concentrations are usually in the upper half of the normal range or hypernatraemic at presentation. This reflects the profound loss of body water as a result of the often prolonged diuresis prior to presentation. The calculations mentioned under investigations for electrolytes in DKA are particularly helpful in estimating plasma sodium levels in HONK, when glucose concentrations are markedly raised.
- **Potassium:** Depletion is also a major feature of HONK although, as with DKA, the plasma potassium at presentation may be low, normal or raised.
- **Urea and creatinine:** Often markedly raised, reflecting severe prerenal impairment.
- **Bicarbonate:** May be slightly low because of lactic acid accumulation resulting from hypotension and poor peripheral tissue blood flow. As the name implies, significant ketoacid accumulation does not occur but patients may show + or + + levels of ketones in their urine. This does not signify DKA.

Treatment

The principles of treatment for HONK are similar to those for DKA, although no controlled trials have been reported. In the following section, some differences in emphasis in the management of HONK compared with DKA will be highlighted.

Fluids and electrolytes

Rehydration is the most important initial treatment and isotonic saline is the fluid of choice. Where dehydration is severe and the patient is hypotensive, sufficient fluid needs to be given to restore blood pressure, and a regimen similar to that suggested for DKA is required. However, with dilution, plasma glucose concentrations fall, and the reduction in osmotic pressure causes fluid to shift to the extravascular and intracellular compartments. Consequently, serum sodium concentrations often increase during early treatment, and, if it is >150 mmol/litre, 0.45% saline should be used as the principal rehydration fluid.

Once an adequate blood pressure has been restored, rehydration can be continued with a view to restoring the fluid deficit over the following 48-72 hours. A slower rehydration regimen is recommended in treating severe HONK, partly to allow time for fluid shifts between intravascular, extravascular and intracellular compartments, and partly because most patients are elderly with coexisting cardiovascular or renal disease.

Insulin

The lack of severe acidosis in HONK, and the effects of rehydration alone in lowering blood glucose at a rate of 3–5 mmol/h, mean that less insulin is needed early in treatment. Patients with HONK are more sensitive to the hypoglycaemic effects of insulin, and rapid falls of blood glucose may occur if high infusion rates are chosen. An infusion rate of 1–2 units/h of insulin should be started, if blood glucose concentrations do not fall with rehydration, adjusted to maintain a rate of fall of blood glucose of 3–5 mmol/h.

Anticoagulation

The risk of arterial and venous thromboses is greater in HONK than in DKA and, providing there is no contraindication, patients should receive full anticoagulation with heparin until they have recovered and are mobile.

Follow-up

Full recovery from a severe episode of HONK may take several days and, in particular, the plasma sodium may not return to the normal range for over a week. Once patients are able to eat and drink, intravenous fluids and insulin can be stopped and the patient provided with a low refined carbohydrate diet. Adequate glycaemic control can sometimes be achieved with simple diet alone, but it may be necessary to continue twice daily insulin treatment for a few weeks until the patient has fully recovered. It is important to consider withdrawing insulin treatment under supervision after this time since, in the long term, insulin is seldom necessary to maintain diabetic control.

Lactic acidosis

Lactate is the primary product of tissue glycolysis and it is usually recycled by the liver into glucose (the Cori cycle). Normal plasma concentrations are 0.6–1.2 mmol/litre. Physiological increases of blood lactate may be >10 mmol/litre during anaerobic metabolism in severe exercise, but this is cleared rapidly by the liver. Pathologically, lactate may accumulate in a variety of disease states whether or not diabetes is present (Table 3.12). Since the initial product of metabolism is lactic acid, for every lactate produced a hydrogen ion is also released into the circulation resulting in a metabolic acidosis.

Table 3.12   Classification of causes of lactic acidosis

Classification	Mechanism	Causes
Type A	Poor tissue perfusion	Cardiogenic shock
		Haemorrhagic shock
		Septicaemic shock
		Post-grand mal seizure
Type B1	Disease-associated	Chronic liver disease
B2	Drug-associated	Biguanides in type 2 diabetes
		Alcohol
		Methanol/ethylene glycol
B3	Inborn errors of metabolism	Rare metabolic myopathies

Because of the increased risk of ischaemic heart disease and cardiogenic shock, patients with diabetes are at greater risk of Type A lactic acidosis, but the underlying cause is usually clinically obvious. Type A lactic acidosis may also occur in patients with DKA as a result of severe dehydration. The raised lactate, which may occasionally be >5 mmol/litre, contributes to the metabolic acidosis.

Type B2 lactic acidosis occurs in type 2 diabetes as a result of biguanide therapy. In a review of 330 cases of biguanide-related lactic acidosis, 281 cases resulted from phenformin, 30 from buformin and 12 from metformin. Phenformin was withdrawn during the 1970s and buformin earlier. Metformin, the only currently available biguanide, is rarely associated with lactic acidosis, providing it is avoided in patients with chronic renal, liver or heart failure (see Chapter 2). Clinical features of lactic acidosis are shown in Table 3.13, and it should be suspected in a severely ill diabetic patient with a metabolic acidosis and absence of ketonuria.

Table 3.13   Clinical features of lactic acidosis

Symptom	Prevalence (%)
Vomiting	52
Impairment of consciousness	50
Nausea	36
Epigastric pain	35
Loss of appetite	26
Overbreathing	25
Lethargy	15
Diarrhoea	13

The anion gap, calculated as:

$$[\text{plasma } (Na^+) + \text{plasma } (K^+)] - [(\text{plasma } (Cl^-) + \text{plasma } (HCO^-_3)]$$

should normally be 14 ± 4 mmol/litre. In lactic acidosis, this will be much higher. Definitive diagnosis requires measurement of blood lactate which is usually >5 mmol/litre, and may be of some benefit in prognosis. Levels >10 mmol/litre are associated with a mortality in excess of 50%.

Treatment of lactic acidosis is empirical. With severe acidosis (pH<7.0) infusion of isotonic sodium bicarbonate, typically 500–1000 mmol during the first 24 hours, with arterial pH monitoring, has been the mainstay of treatment,[14] although there is no controlled trial evidence to support this approach. Correction of dehydration and hypoxia are also important. Coexistent diabetes should be controlled with continuous infusion of dextrose and insulin.

References

1 Faich GA, Fishbein HA, Ellis SE. The epidemiology of diabetic ketoacidosis; a population based study. *Am J Epidemiol* 1983;**117**: 551.

2 Johnson DD, Palumbo PJ, Chu CP. Diabetic ketoacidosis in a community-based population. *Mayo Clinic Proc* 1980;**55**:83–8.

3 Tunbridge WMG. Factors contributing to the deaths of diabetics under 50 years of age. *Lancet* 1981;**i**:569–72.

4 Chapman J, Wright AD, Nattran M *et al.* Recurrent diabetic ketoacidosis. *Diabetic Med* 1985;**5**;659–61.

5 Mecklenburg RS, Benson EA, Benson JW Jr *et al.* Acute complications associated with insulin infusion pump therapy. *J Am Med Ass* 1984; **252**:3265–9.

6 Chauhan SP, Perry KG Jr. Management of diabetic ketoacidosis in the obstetric patient. *Obstet Gynecol Clin N Amer* 1995;**22**:143–55.

7 Beigelman PM. Potassium in severe diabetic ketoacidosis. *Am J Med* 1974;**54**:419–20.

8 Alberti KGMM. Low dose insulin in the treatment of diabetic ketoacidosis. *Arch Intern Med* 1977;**137**:1367–76.

9 Barrett EJ, DeFronzo RA, Bevilacqua S, Ferrannini E. Insulin resistance in diabetic ketoacidosis. *Diabetes* 1982;**31**:923–8.

10 Lever E, Jaspan JB. Sodium bicarbonate therapy in severe diabetic ketoacidosis. *Am J Med* 1983;**75**:263–8.

11 Dorman JS, LaPorte RE, Kuller LH. The Pittsburgh insulin-dependent diabetes mellitus morbidity and mortality study. II Mortality results. *Diabetes* 1984;**33**:271–6.

12 Rosenbloom AL. Intracerebral crises during treatment of diabetic ketoacidosis. *Diabetes Care* 1990;**13**:1–32.

13 Grant C, Warlow C. Focal epilepsy in diabetic nonketotic hyperglycaemia. *Br Med J* 1985;**290**:1204–5.

14 Mizock BA. Controversies in the management of lactic acidosis. *J Am Med Ass* 1987;**258**:497–501.

4 Hypoglycaemia

A&E departments treat most episodes of hypoglycaemia that reach hospital, but an understanding of the causes, diagnosis and treatment is necessary in many other departments. For example, hypoglycaemia may be seen on surgical wards as a result of pre- and postoperative changes to insulin or sulphonylurea therapy, in obstetric practice because of tight antenatal glycaemic control, and in neurology outpatients, where a patient with type 1 diabetes may be referred for investigation of seizures.

Definitions

Hypoglycaemia can be defined in several ways:

- *Biochemical*: when the plasma glucose falls below an arbitrary value (2.8 mmol/litre)
- *Clinical*: associated with symptoms or signs; it can be further divided into:
  - *mild*: identified and treated by the patient
  - *severe*: the patient requires the assistance of another person
  - *coma*: self-explanatory.

How common is hypoglycaemia?

Type 1 diabetes

Mild hypoglycaemia is part of the daily lives in many of these patients, and is seen as an inevitable but not particularly threatening nuisance. A Danish survey of over 400 patients, most of whom used twice daily insulin regimens, reported an average of two mild episodes per patient each week with more occurring during workdays than weekends.[1]

The prevalence of severe hypoglycaemia can be summarised using the "rule of thirds", suggested by Gale (Box 4.1).[2]

> # Box 4.1 Rule of thirds for severe hypoglycaemia
>
> - One in three patients (30%) will experience a hypoglycaemic coma during their diabetic lifetime, of whom
> - One in three (10%) will have experienced a hypoglycaemic coma in the last year, of whom
> - One in three (2–3%) will have recurrent severe hypoglycaemia which disrupts their lives

In the Danish survey, severe hypoglycaemia with coma was reported in 36% of patients during their diabetic lifetime, and 10% had experienced more than 10 episodes of coma. Similar data, suggesting an incidence of severe hypoglycaemia of about 10% per year, have been reported from other European countries, America, Canada and New Zealand. A striking feature of the Danish survey was that only 5% of patients were treated in hospital, most episodes being dealt with by relatives, friends or work colleagues. Although A&E departments see only the tip of the iceberg, a few patients with recurrent episodes can be responsible for a significant number of attendances. In a one-year survey at a large A&E department, 200 admissions resulting from hypoglycaemia were identified: 96 had one admission whilst 34 patients were admitted on 104 occasions. Average insulin doses in those with recurrent admissions were higher than in a matched population, suggesting that over-treatment was an important cause.[3]

Hypoglycaemia risk is related to the intensity of diabetes control (Figure 4.1). In the intensively treated arm of the Diabetes Control and Complications Trial, the incidence increased three-fold to 62 episodes per 100 patient years.[4]

Type 2 diabetes

In the UK Prospective Diabetes Survey, mild hypoglycaemia was reported in 37% of patients on insulin after three years, and 2.3% had experienced a severe attack needing third party assistance, suggesting an incidence of 2.3% per year compared with 10% per year for type 1 diabetes.[5]

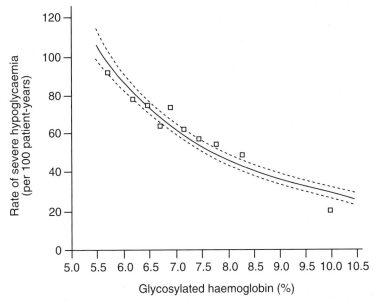

Figure 4.1   Rate of severe hypoglycaemia in patients receiving intensive therapy, according to their mean glycosylated haemoglobin values during the trial. The mean of the monthly values was used. Squares indicate the crude rates within deciles of the mean glycosylated haemoglobin values during the trial; each square corresponds to more than 400 patient years. The solid lines are regression lines estimated as a function of the log of the glycosylated haemoglobin values. The dashed lines are 95% confidence intervals. (with permission of New England Journal of Medicine[4]).

Hypoglycaemia may also occur in people taking sulphonylureas. Estimates of the risk vary, but one survey reported that 20% of patients experienced mild symptoms during six months' treatment with sulphonylureas.[6] This has been confirmed by the UK Prospective Diabetes Survey in which 17% of patients on sulphonylureas experienced mild clinical hypoglycaemia per year. Severe episodes are much less common than in people with either type 1 diabetes or insulin-treated type 2 diabetes, with an incidence of 0.25/1000 people per year.

Pathophysiology

The brain cannot store glucose and is critically dependent on a continuous supply from the circulation. It is defended by several homeostatic mechanisms that maintain blood glucose within a narrow range in health. These can be classified under two headings:

79

- Euglycaemic counterregulation.
- Hypoglycaemic counterregulation.

Euglycaemic counterregulation

In healthy subjects, blood glucose is prevented from falling during short-term fasting (e.g. overnight) by hepatic glucose production from glycogen breakdown and gluconeogenesis. Changes in the ratio of insulin and glucagon in portal blood regulate hepatic glucose production, with fasting being associated with suppression of insulin and stimulation of glucagon secretion.

Hypoglycaemic counterregulation

People treated with insulin or sulphonylureas cannot "switch off" insulin in the presence of falling blood glucose concentrations and, as a result of continued glucose uptake by peripheral tissues and reduced hepatic glucose production, are at risk of hypo-glycaemia. The brain "senses" impending hypoglycaemia and activates neuroendocrine counterregulatory responses which counteract it (Figure 4.2).

Two counterregulatory hormones, glucagon and adrenaline, are of central importance in the acute defence against hypoglycaemia. Glucagon transiently increases glycogenolysis and causes a more sustained increase in gluconeogenesis, thereby increasing glucose output from the liver to the systemic circulation. Adrenaline also stimulates hepatic glucose production, but also inhibits glucose disposal in peripheral tissues.

Their relative importance in counterregulation has been studied by pharmacologically inhibiting each of the hormones and measuring the effect on insulin-induced hypoglycaemia. These studies show that:

- Inhibition of glucagon (and growth hormone) by somatostatin reduces blood glucose recovery by about 40%.
- Inhibition of adrenergic responses with alpha and beta blockade, in the presence of a normal glucagon response does not interfere with glucose recovery.
- A combination of inhibition of glucagon and adrenergic blockade causes a profound defect in glucose recovery.

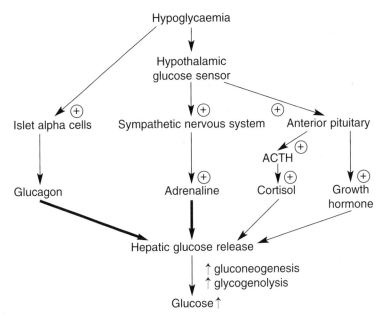

Figure 4.2 Hypoglycaemia counterregulatory mechanisms.

It can be concluded from the above that in normal subjects glucagon is the principal defence against hypoglycaemia, and adrenaline acts as a "backup" in the event of glucagon deficiency.

Cortisol and growth hormone both inhibit glucose disposal in peripheral tissues and induce the expression of key enzymes in the gluconeogenic pathway but, because these effects take several hours to become manifest, neither hormone is important in acute counterregulation. Deficiency of either or both, as occurs in panhypopituitarism, results in increased sensitivity to insulin and slightly delayed recovery to hypoglycaemia, suggesting an important permissive role of both hormones in prolonged hypoglycaemia.

Symptoms and signs

Symptoms of hypoglycaemia can be broadly divided into three groups:

- autonomic
- neuroglycopaenic
- non-specific.

81

Box 4.2 expands on these groups.

Box 4.2 Symptoms and signs of hypoglycaemia

- *Autonomic*
  - Sweating
  - Tremor
  - Pounding heart
  - Anxiety
  - Hunger

- *Neuroglycopaenic*
  - Confusion
  - Odd behaviour
  - Inability to concentrate
  - Drowsiness
  - Visual disturbance
  - Tingling around mouth

- *Non-specific*
  - Weakness
  - Dizziness
  - Headache
  - Parasthesiae

Autonomic symptoms are a direct result of activation of the sympathetic nervous system together with the release of adrenaline from the adrenal medulla. In non-diabetic subjects the threshold for autonomic symptoms is a blood glucose of 2.8–3.2 mmol/litre (Figure 4.3). Recognition of autonomic symptoms should warn someone of impending hypoglycaemia and allow appropriate action to be taken.

One problem for people with diabetes in recognising impending hypoglycaemia is that cerebral function begins to deteriorate with blood glucose concentrations above the threshold for autonomic activation, if this threshold is lowered by overtight glycaemic control.

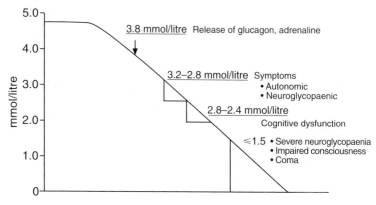

Figure 4.3   Glycaemic thresholds for onset of symptoms of acute hypoglycaemia in non-diabetic subjects.

Neuroglycopaenic symptoms vary markedly between people but tend to be constant for each individual. Early symptoms may include a feeling of light-headedness, tingling around the mouth and vacant feeling. As blood glucose falls further, movements may become slow, the speech slurred and coordination poor. Irritability or uncharacteristic aggression are common and such changes in behaviour are often first recognised by relatives or friends. Automatism may occur in which patients continue to perform complex tasks, such as driving with no awareness of their actions and no recall of events afterwards.

With increasingly severe hypoglycaemia, drowsiness and eventual coma develop which, if prolonged, can lead to irreversible brain injury.

Severe neuroglycopaenia can also result in:

- **Convulsions**: About 10% of episodes of severe hypoglycaemia in adults and 22–37% in children may be associated with generalised grand mal seizures. The occurrence of seizures in a patient with type 1 diabetes may lead to an incorrect diagnosis of epilepsy. All such episodes should be considered due to hypoglycaemia until proved otherwise. Measurement of the blood glucose during or soon after a seizure will confirm hypoglycaemia as the precipitant but this is often not possible. Several other clinical features may provide indirect evidence (Box 4.3). Adjustment of insulin dose, regimen or diet is required where hypoglycaemia is shown to be responsible for seizures. If the problem is one of nocturnal seizures, a useful tip is to ask patients to test their blood before going to bed. A result <7 mmol/litre is associated with a greater risk of nocturnal hypoglycaemia and should prompt the patient to have a carbohydrate snack.

Box 4.3 Clinical pointers to hypoglycaemia as a cause of seizures

- Excessive insulin doses or inappropriate insulin regimen
- Normal or low HBA_{1c} values suggesting tight diabetic control
- Seizures occurring at high risk times for hypoglycaemia (e.g. 2.00–6.00 am)
- Direct evidence of hypoglycaemia on routine home blood glucose testing

---

- **Hemiplegia**: This is a rare manifestation of hypoglycaemia that usually occurs in the early hours or on waking. Symptoms usually resolve "on the end of the needle" but occasionally recovery may take several hours. There is obvious potential for misdiagnosis of hemiplegic hypoglycaemia for a cerebrovascular event, and it is important to check a laboratory blood glucose in any person with diabetes with sudden onset of focal neurological signs.

Causes of hypoglycaemia

The main precipitants of hypoglycaemia in patients with type 1 diabetes are:

- **Excessive doses of insulin**: Will inevitably be associated with an increased risk of hypoglycaemia. A number of other factors influence the rate of insulin absorption from injection sites and may increase the risk (Table 4.1).

Table 4.1   Factors influencing insulin absorption rate from injection sites

Mechanism	Comment
Changing site of injection	Absorption rates: abdomen>arms>thigh
Skin temperature	Hypoglycaemia after hot bath or sauna
Lipohypertrophy	Erratic absorption of insulin
Inadvertent intramuscular injection	Rapid absorption

- **Delayed or missed meals**: A depot of subcutaneous insulin will continue to act whether or not the patient has eaten. With twice daily regimens of short- and intermediate-acting insulin, risk is greatest late morning particularly if lunch is delayed, or between midnight and 4.00 am. Alcohol is an important contributory factor which masks the warning symptoms or impairs the patient's ability to take appropriate action. Surveys in A&E departments suggest that up to 20% of episodes of hypoglycaemia are associated with alcohol.
- **Exercise**: Increases the rate of insulin absorption from subcutaneous tissues and improves peripheral insulin action. Where exercise is planned, many patients reduce their insulin dose or have extra carbohydrate, but since the insulin-sensitising effect of exercise can last up to 18 hours, hypoglycaemia can occur the following morning after a game of squash.[7]

Who is most at risk?

A number of physiological and pathophysiological changes increase the risk of hypoglycaemia in type 1 diabetes which can be considered under the following headings.

Impaired counterregulation (hypoglycaemic unawareness)

"Overtight" diabetic control

There are two reasons why warning symptoms may be reduced in patients with overtight diabetic control. First, an episode of hypoglycaemia impairs the counterregulatory hormone responses to further episodes for at least a week. Secondly, frequent mild episodes, which are common in patients with tight diabetic control, lower the threshold at which the sympathetic nervous system is activated. As a result, such patients increasingly rely on neuroglycopaenic symptoms to identify an impending attack, with a greater risk of severe neuroglycopaenia.

An intensive training programme with avoidance of hypoglycaemia by regular blood glucose testing and regular snacks between meals may restore counterregulatory hormone responses and lead to a return of hypoglycaemic warning symptoms (Figure 4.4).[8]

Type 1 diabetes of long duration

One in three patients with type 1 diabetes for over 20 years has reduced warning symptoms of hypoglycaemia. Sweating and tremor become less marked and patients have to rely much more on neuroglycopaenic symptoms to recognise impending hypoglycaemia. Symptoms may also develop more quickly. Reduced counterregulatory hormone responses are partly responsible for these changes in warning symptoms (Figure 4.5). After five years most patients have an impaired glucagon response to hypoglycaemia and depend much more on adrenergic "back-up". After 15 or more years adrenaline responses are also impaired in up to 40% of patients with a consequent delay in restoration of normoglycaemia.

Beta-blockers

Non-selective beta-blockers, such as propranolol, delay the recovery from hypoglycaemia. This may be particularly marked

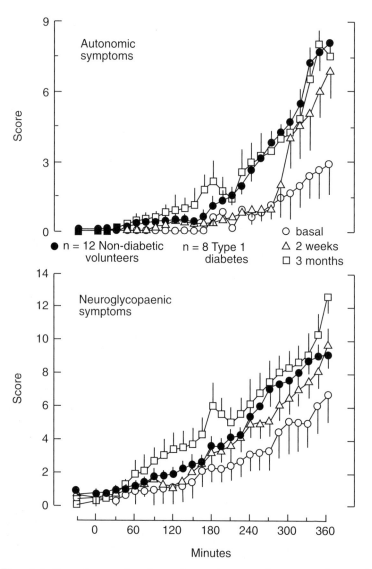

Figure 4.4 Score of autonomic and neuroglycopaenic symptoms' responses to the stepped hypoglycaemia in non-diabetic volunteer subjects and type 1 diabetes patients, studied at baseline, after two weeks and three months of meticulous prevention of hypoglycaemia (with permission of Diabetes[8]*).*

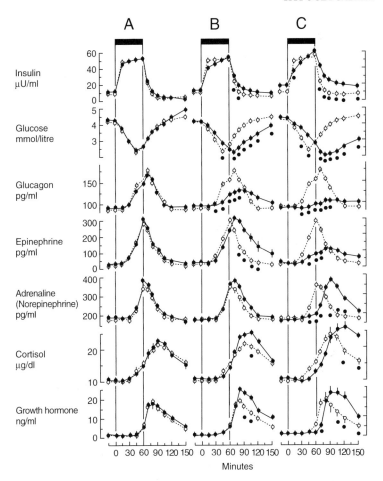

Figure 4.5 Plasma insulin, glucose, and counterregulatory hormone concentrations in response to insulin-induced hypolycaemia in diabetic subjects (●—●) and in 10 non-diabetic subjects (○--○). Insulin was infused from 0 through 60 minutes (28 mU/m²/min). Diabetic patients were rendered euglycaemic by overnight i.v. infusion of insulin, and the basal insulin infusion rate required to maintain euglycaemia from − 60 to 0 minutes was continued through 60 minutes (A, group A: five diabetic patients, diabetes duration <1 month; B, group B: 11 diabetic patients, diabetes duration 1–5 years; C, group C: five diabetic patients, duration of diabetes 14–31 years). *P<0.05, diabetics vs non-diabetics. (With permission from Diabetes.[9]*)*

in those with established glucagon deficiency. Some autonomic symptoms, such as sweating, which is mediated through cholinergic pathways are unaffected by beta-blockade. Cardioselective beta-blockers do not impair glucose recovery from hypoglycaemia and are preferred if beta-blockade is necessary on clinical grounds.

Secondary diabetes

People whose diabetes results from total pancreatectomy or chronic pancreatitis are susceptible to prolonged and severe episodes of hypoglycaemia. This is partly due to impaired counter-regulation because of the absence of pancreatic glucagon. In many such patients alcohol dependency contributes to the initial pancreatic problems, and continued alcohol abuse may be an additional risk factor for severe hypoglycaemia in some patients.

Changes in insulin requirements

Honeymoon period

Control of hyperglycaemia with insulin in a newly diagnosed person with type 1 diabetes results in a return of limited pancreatic endocrine function. This often causes a fall in insulin requirements after six weeks to three months, and advice will be needed on insulin dose reduction if symptomatic hypoglycaemia is to be avoided.

Changing insulin species

Animal insulins stimulate production of insulin antibodies which may prolong the half-life of injected insulin. Transfer to human insulin (especially from beef) usually results in a fall in insulin antibody titre and increased availability of insulin. An initial dose reduction of 10–20% overall is recommended when people are switched from animal to human insulin to lessen the risk of hypoglycaemia. Changing from pork insulin does not need such a large reduction.

Worsening renal function

Insulin requirements decrease with worsening renal function and, unless anticipated in management, may cause hypoglycaemia as is shown in the following case.

Case Study 10

A 57-year-old man with long-standing type 1 diabetes, complicated by retinopathy and diabetic nephropathy, complained of headaches and a "hung over" feeling on waking, which improved after breakfast; he remained well during the day. His insulin regimen (premixed 30/70 preparation, 18 units each morning and 12 units each evening) had been unchanged for several years, but over the last two years his serum creatinine had risen to 355 μmol/litre. His HBA$_{1c}$ had fallen from 8 to 5.6% over the same time. Reduction in his insulin dose to 14 units each morning and 8 units each evening prevented further morning headaches, which were certainly due to hypoglycaemia.

The kidneys catabolise 30–40% of insulin. With advancing renal failure, insulin requirements usually fall. Progressive anorexia and loss of lean body weight also reduce insulin requirements, and insulin doses should be reduced according to blood monitoring results and HBA$_{1c}$ data.

Coincidental endocrine disease

Deficiency of counterregulatory hormones increases the risk of hypoglycaemia as is shown in the following case.

Case Study 11

A 47-year-old woman with long-standing type 1 diabetes had been stable for 15 years on 24 units 30/70 premixed insulin each morning and 16 units each evening. Over six months she had become increasingly tired, and had had two episodes of abdominal pain, vomiting, and diarrhoea. During this period she had several severe hypos and had reduced her total insulin dose by 30%. She was admitted with a further episode of vomiting and abdominal pain, when her electrolytes were Na+ 126 mmol/litre, K+5.8 mmol/litre, urea 12.4 mmol/litre. A diagnosis of Addison's disease was confirmed by a Synacthen test. She improved markedly with intravenous and then oral hydrocortisone together with fludrocortisone. Her daily insulin dose increased and hypoglycaemia was no longer a problem.

Addison's disease is more common in people with type 1 diabetes. Progressive loss of cortisol reserve leads to an increased risk of hypoglycaemia. Other endocrine disorders that increase sensitivity to insulin include hypopituitarism (owing to a combination of cortisol and growth hormone deficiency) and hypothyroidism.

Malabsorption

Coeliac disease is more common in people with type 1 diabetes and may predispose to hypoglycaemia owing to unpredictable

89

small intestinal glucose absorption. Measurement of antigliadin antibodies can be used as a screening test, but endoscopic duodenal biopsy is required if there is a high degree of clinical suspicion.

At-risk patient groups

Children

Small children, especially those under 6 years, because of their unpredictable eating habits and marked variability of physical activity, are at risk of hypoglycaemia. In children under 5 years of age, episodes of hypoglycaemia may be harmful to the developing brain, and targets for glycaemic control should be less strict in this age group. As a matter of course, parents need to be taught how to recognise hypoglycaemia, which presents with different symptoms, mainly behavioural, and how to treat it.

Pregnancy

The objective of very strict glycaemic control in diabetic pregnancy makes hypoglycaemia more likely, since it is also associated with a blunting of warning symptoms. There is no evidence that acute hypoglycaemia is teratogenic, although prolonged episodes with precipitation of seizures are undesirable for fetal development. Sudden, frequent hypoglycaemic episodes in the third trimester, reflecting lower insulin resistance, may occasionally result from an intrauterine death, but this is not a particularly reliable clinical feature. Immediately post-delivery, insulin requirements fall to prepregnancy levels, and patients need to resume their pre-pregnancy doses, rather than those used in the third trimester, to avoid severe postnatal hypoglycaemia. Women who breast-feed often find they need to reduce their insulin doses by 10–20% to allow for the carbohydrate transferred to breast milk.

Frequent blood glucose monitoring and insulin dose adjustment are essential to minimise the risk, but patients and their partners should be provided with glucagon for use in emergencies and shown how to use it.

The elderly

The elderly can be vulnerable to hypoglycaemia because of erratic meal patterns and errors in insulin administration as is shown in the following case.

Case Study 12

An 84-year-old lady was admitted, having been found semi-conscious by her home help. She had long-standing type 1 diabetes controlled with two injections of premixed 30/70 insulin each day. Hypoglycaemia was confirmed in hospital, and she improved with intravenous glucose. Over the next 12 hours she had two further episodes, and a continuous glucose infusion was started.

She could not remember how much insulin she had injected on the day of admission. A Diabetes Nurse Specialist watched her draw up (unsuccessfully) and give a test injection. She was transferred to once-daily insulin and arrangements were made for the district nurse to call on her daily to draw up and give the injection.

Some elderly patients have difficulties drawing up and administering insulin. The reasons are many and varied, but include poor vision due to retinopathy, cataract or senile macular degeneration, arthritis, or tremor. Impairment of memory can lead to injections being omitted or given twice. Sometimes the loss of a partner who had previously assumed responsibility for supervising treatment can precipitate a series of diabetic admissions in a vulnerable patient, so called "brittle diabetes of the elderly". The following case is illustrative.

Case Study 13

A 75-year-old lady with a 20-year history of type 1 diabetes was admitted to casualty with diabetic ketoacidosis. There had been no previous admissions with uncontrolled diabetes. She had attended a hospital diabetes clinic regularly and had maintained reasonably good diabetic control. Several entries in the medical notes referred to her poor understanding of diabetes management, and she was unable to name the type of insulin she was using. She had always attended clinic appointments with her husband who had recently died.

She recovered with standard treatment, no precipitating cause was identified, and she was discharged with outpatient follow-up. Over the following six months she had two further admissions with ketoacidosis and one with hypoglycaemia. It became clear that she had depended on her husband for supervision of her diabetes, and with his death she was unable to cope. The situation was finally resolved when she agreed to move into sheltered accommodation where she could be supervised.

Sulphonylurea-related hypoglycaemia

Hypoglycaemia associated with the sulphonylureas is less common than in patients treated with insulin but is more likely to be fatal. The annual incidence has been reported as 19 per 1000 patient years for all episodes and 0.25 per 1000 patient years for severe episodes associated with coma. A number of factors increase the risk of sulphonylurea-induced hypoglycaemia (Box 4.4).

Box 4.4 Factors increasing the risk of sulphonylurea-induced hypoglycaemia

- Increasing age
- Restricted food intake
- Impaired renal function
- Impaired hepatic function

The elderly are at particular risk. In a Swedish Adverse Drug Reaction Registry survey of 57 episodes, the 10 deaths all occurred in patients over 75 years of age who were taking glibenclamide.[10] The severity of hypoglycaemia was not confined to patients taking large doses, and as little as 2.5 mg/day could be fatal. Various sulphonylureas have been apportioned different relative risks of inducing hypoglycaemia depending on their potency, route of elimination and half-life (Table 4.2).

Table 4.2 Route of elimination, half-life and relative hypoglycaemic potential of common sulphonylureas

Drug	Route of metabolism	Plasma half-life (h)	Relative risk
Tolbutamide	Liver (inactive metabolites)	6–12	1.0
Glipizide	Liver (inactive metabolites)	3–7	2.2
Gliclazide	Liver (inactive metabolites)	10–12	2.0
Glibenclamide	Liver (inactive metabolites)	10–16	4.8
Chlorpromamide	Renal (excreted unchanged)	24–40	5.3

Sulphonylurea-induced hypoglycaemia can be insidious in onset, and may present as progressive cognitive impairment, or focal neurological symptoms suggesting a transient ischaemic attack or established stroke. **Hypoglycaemia should be considered in any**

patient on sulphonylureas who presents with a disturbance of cerebral function.

Worsening renal function can also increase the risk of hypoglycaemia in those on sulphonylureas; the following case illustrates this.

Case Study 14

A 74-year-old man was referred by his general practitioner with several weeks of malaise and altered behaviour, which was initially diagnosed as a viral illness. He had become much worse on the day of admission and was unable to give any account of himself. He was described as "looking very vacant". He had had type 2 diabetes since 1980 and had been well controlled on diet and glibenclamide 5 mg/day for over 10 years. Renal impairment was first noted in 1987 when he had an elective repair of an aortic aneurysm; his creatinine had risen gradually to 527 μmol/litre. Investigations two years earlier had confirmed this was due to hypertensive and ischaemic renal disease rather than diabetic nephropathy.

Blood glucose on admission was 1.4 mmol/litre and he was treated with 25% dextrose. Over the following three days, despite stopping his glibenclamide, he needed a continuous infusion of 5% and later 10% dextrose to prevent further episodes. In this situation, infusing glucose may make matters worse by further stimulating insulin secretion. The somatostatin analogue, octreotide (50–100 μg tds by s.c. injection), directly inhibits insulin release from the beta-cells, and was successful in stabilising the patient's blood glucose. He was eventually stabilised on diet alone.

The long half-life of some sulphonylureas can also cause problems in postoperative patients on surgical wards and the potential for recurrent severe hypoglycaemia may not be recognised, as is illustrated in the next case.

Case Study 15

An elderly man was admitted for an elective cholecystectomy. He had type 2 diabetes, controlled with diet and glibenclamide 10 mg/day. On the day of surgery his oral hypoglycaemic medication had been withheld, and he underwent surgery early on the morning list. His early postoperative ward capillary blood glucose results had been in the range of 7–12 mmol/litre and he was prescribed 0.9% saline with potassium to be given at a rate of 100 ml/h. He was not able to eat supper.

During the early part of the night he was noted to be unwell with slurring of his speech, confusion, and disorientation. Capillary

93

blood glucose had fallen to 1.7 mmol/litre and he was treated with an intravenous injection of 25 ml of 25% dextrose by the duty house surgeon. The patient improved and was settled for the night by nursing staff with no instructions to repeat the glucose measurement during the night. The following morning he was found comatose with a glucose of 1.3 mmol/litre, and it took several days before his cerebral function returned to normal.

The message underlying these cases is that hypoglycaemia caused by long-acting sulphonylureas is potentially life-threatening and usually requires hospital admission for up to 72 hours. Patients on sulphonylureas who are unable to eat for any reason require regular blood glucose monitoring for up to 72 hours even if the drug is discontinued.

Concomitant drug therapy can potentiate the hypoglycaemic effects of sulphonylureas, although the prevalence of such events is unknown. Examples are shown in Table 4.3.

Table 4.3   Drug interactions with sulphonylureas increasing risk of hypoglycaemia

Mechanism	Examples
Reduced plasma protein binding	Warfarin, fibrates, salicylates
Reduced hepatic metabolism	Warfarin, chloramphenicol
Increased insulin secretion	NSAIDs
Decreased renal excretion	Salicylates
Increased peripheral glucose uptake	Salicylates

Table 4.4   Treatment of hypoglycaemia

Duration of hypoglycaemia	Treatment of choice	Next best
Minutes		
Patient	Oral CHO	Glucagon 1 mg
Relative	Oral CHO (liquid/solid)	
Hours		
Primary care team Paramedics	Glucagon 1 mg	25 g dextrose i.v.
A&E department	25 g dextrose i.v.	Glucagon 1 mg

CHO = carbohydrate

Treatment

The first priority in treating hypoglycaemia is returning blood glucose to normal as quickly as possible. Treatment should be tailored to the severity and duration of the hypoglycaemia (Box 4.5 and Table 4.4).

Box 4.5 Treatment options for hypoglycaemia

- Oral carbohydrate >20 g as Dextrosol tablets (3.1 g/tablet)
- Buccal carbohydrate as Hypostop or Lucozade
- Glucagon 1 mg (subcutaneous, intramuscular or intravenous)
- Intravenous dextrose 25 g, 50 ml of 50% dextrose

Oral therapy

Mild symptoms

Mild hypoglycaemia is a common experience of many patients on insulin and a smaller proportion on sulphonylureas. Such episodes are usually short-lived, since most patients will recognise warning symptoms and take extra carbohydrate. Providing it is palatable, rapidly absorbed, and convenient, the type of carbohydrate used is less important. Many diabetes clinics recommend 3 Dextrosol tablets (9.3 g total CHO), repeated after five minutes if symptoms persist, but other forms of refined carbohydrate, such as digestive biscuits or sandwiches, are equally effective.

Mild hypoglycaemia is common in patients on medical or surgical wards. The principles of management are similar, but patients may not have access to carbohydrate in the ward or may be unable to take it. Medical and nursing staff need to be alert to the risk of hypoglycaemia. Patients who can eat should be encouraged to have glucose tablets or a suitable alternative on their bedside locker. Clear guidelines need to be given to nursing staff for those patients who are unable to eat.

Severe attacks

Most episodes are treated in the community by relatives, work colleagues, or by primary care or emergency services. Several treatment options are available, and medical staff dealing with

95

cases that reach hospital should try to provide appropriate advice on the best ways of preventing future episodes. Sometimes this information will need to be followed up by diabetes nurse specialists. The options available for treatment by mouth are:

- *Glucose in liquid form:* Patients who are unable to take glucose by mouth or who are uncooperative can be effectively treated with preparations of liquid glucose such as Lucozade (19.3 g/ 100 ml). Relatives often recognise impending severe hypoglycaemia by changes in behaviour, and some patients become uncooperative and reluctant to accept advice. Firm encouragement is sometimes needed to persuade a hypoglycaemic patient to take a glucose drink even if it is initially refused. It may be necessary to pour glucose liquid into the patient's mouth providing they are conscious, although Lucozade can be easily spat out or aspirated into the trachea.
- *Glucose paste (Hypostop):* Hypostop is a glucose gel solution containing 32 g/100 ml. It is supplied in a squeezable plastic bottle with a flexible tube for administration into the buccal cavity of an uncooperative semiconscious patient, where it melts, trickles into the oesophagus, and is swallowed. It can be particularly useful in children.
- All glucose-based drinks or gel preparations are short-lived, and there is a risk of further hypoglycaemia after 30 minutes or so. Patients should **always** be encouraged to have longer acting carbohydrate, such as sandwiches, on recovery.

Parenteral therapy

Two parenteral forms of treatment for hypoglycaemia are available:

Glucagon

Glucagon increases blood glucose by stimulating glycogen breakdown in the liver. It is supplied as a powder which has to be reconstituted with diluent (supplied by both leading manufacturers) before administration. In this form it has a shelf-life of two years. It works most rapidly when given intravenously but, if this is difficult in an uncooperative patient, it is almost as effective when given intramuscularly or subcutaneously, and restores consciousness in most patients within about 10 minutes.[11] To prevent relapse, patients should take extra carbohydrate by mouth, but this may prove difficult because nausea and vomiting can affect up to one in three patients after glucagon.

Education of patients and, more importantly, their relatives, plays a crucial role in ensuring glucagon is used correctly. Dealing with a semiconscious hypoglycaemic loved one is not the best time to read the package insert! Even with education, some relatives are so paralysed with anxiety that they cannot administer glucagon.

The variety of routes of administration for glucagon is an advantage for paramedics and primary care physicians in dealing with patients who are restless, uncooperative, or fitting. However, where severe hypoglycaemia has been prolonged (>30 min) glucagon is less effective, presumably because of exhaustion of hepatic glycogen by the normal counterregulatory response. Some patients may also respond poorly to glucagon because of reduced glycogen reserves (Box 4.6) and in these circumstances intravenous glucose is the treatment of choice.

Box 4.6 Clinical conditions associated with a poor response to glucagon

- Thin/malnourished
- Alcohol abuse
- Chronic liver disease
- Addison's disease
- Hypopituitarism

Intravenous dextrose

Intravenous dextrose remains the most rapid and effective treatment for a severe attack. It is recommended as first-line treatment in most A&E departments, particularly if glucagon has already been given and has not worked. Comparative studies suggest that intravenous dextrose works slightly more quickly and produces a higher peak of blood glucose than glucagon.[11] A 50 ml dose of 50% dextrose will cause average blood sugar concentrations to increase from 1 to 12.5 mmol/litre, leading to return of a normal level of consciousness within five minutes. If possible, the injection should be given into an antecubital vein to minimise the risk of thrombophlebitis and thrombosis.

What if the patient doesn't wake up?

Most patients with severe hypoglycaemia treated in hospital regain consciousness within minutes of treatment being given, with about 30% having nausea or headache on recovery. A few patients may remain unconscious, and a variety of possible diagnoses should be considered (Box 4.7).

Box 4.7 Differential diagnoses in unconscious patients

- Prolonged hypoglycaemia with cerebral oedema
- Postictal following a hypoglycaemic seizure
- Head injury
- Coincidental intracerebral or subarachnoid haemorrhage
- Drug overdose

This situation demands careful re-evaluation of the patient. The history from an eye witness can be of great help in confirming a seizure or head injury, and physical signs such as pupillary changes, preretinal haemorrhages, or neck stiffness may require an urgent cranial CT scan.

The immediate priority to maintain blood glucose in the range of 7–15 mmol/litre can be achieved with a dextrose infusion and hourly monitoring of capillary blood glucose. With no improvement after four hours, a CT scan should be considered. As well as excluding treatable intracerebral disease, it may confirm cerebral oedema, a recognised complication of prolonged hypoglycaemia. Treatment of hypoglycaemia-related cerebral oedema is essentially supportive. Dexamethasone (4 mg qds), mannitol infusion, and hypocapnoeic positive pressure ventilatory support have all been suggested as management strategies but with no clear evidence of benefit.

Prevention

In the euphoria following revival of a deeply unconscious patient "on the end of the needle", there is a tendency to forget that the treatment has been needed because of a previous treatment failure. Hypoglycaemia is usually an unpleasant and frightening experience for patients, and prevention of future episodes should be part of the management plan. This demands an understanding of why the hypoglycaemia occurred so that appropriate measures can be put in place to minimise future risk. Patients may need adequate education or re-education on the causes and recognition of hypoglycaemia, adjustment of insulin or tablets may be needed, and patients and their relatives should be provided with suitable treatments for future hypoglycaemic emergencies. Patients with long-duration diabetes and impaired awareness of hypoglycaemia are a particularly vulnerable group who usually have to rely heavily on self-monitored blood glucose testing.

Overdoses

Insulin

Literature reports of deliberate insulin overdose certainly underestimate the real number of cases. A survey of deaths in type 1 diabetes patients under 50 years of age in the UK in 1981 recorded hypoglycaemia as the cause in 4%.[12] Of these, several patients had psychiatric histories and were thought to have committed suicide. Most cases occur in patients with type 1 diabetes and associated psychiatric problems, but occasional episodes are seen in close relatives or health professionals who have access to insulin. Doses of between 200 and 3200 units of insulin have been used in reported attempts. Because the peripheral effect of insulin on the glucose transport mechanism is maximal at doses in excess of 200 units of insulin, patients who take larger doses do not experience more severe hypoglycaemia, but require longer periods of support until the insulin is dissipated, particularly if longer-acting preparations have been used.

Treatment of a large insulin overdose is straightforward and requires infusion of sufficient glucose intravenously to maintain blood glucose concentrations at or above normal. The maximum amount of glucose which can be taken up by peripheral muscle is approximately 50–75 μmol/kg/min. Roughly calculated, this is equivalent to 3.5–4.5 mmol of glucose per minute or 5000 mmol/24 h.

To avoid excessive fluid volume, high concentration glucose infusions (10 or 20%) should be used via a central line or antecubital vein. Care should always be taken to avoid extravasation of such hypertonic fluid into subcutaneous tissues, since this may result in a severe local thrombophlebitis with tissue necrosis. Infusions are usually required for between 24 and 72 hours according to the dose and type of insulin used in the attempt, and regular monitoring of the blood glucose concentration and electrolytes is vital.

Hypokalaemia is a predictable complication of insulin overdose and results from the action of insulin to stimulate potassium uptake by skeletal muscle. Where it occurs, 20 or 40 mmol potassium should be added to the intravenous glucose infusion and the dose adjusted according to laboratory monitoring.

Malicious insulin overdose

Rarely, insulin may be used maliciously by family members or medical staff. The possibility should be considered when hypoglycaemia occurs unexpectedly, for example in a non-diabetic relative of a diabetic patient, or in a nursing home resident, or hospital patient. Under these circumstances, it is essential that a blood sample for measurement of glucose, insulin **and** C-peptide is taken before hypoglycaemia is treated. Hypoglycaemia due to an insulinoma, the important differential diagnosis, will have low-glucose, and high-insulin and C-peptide levels, whereas malicious insulin administration will have low-glucose, high-insulin and low-C-peptide levels.

Sulphonylurea

Deliberate or inadvertent overdose with sulphonylureas is uncommon but can result in severe and sometimes fatal refractory hypoglycaemia. Hypoglycaemia may last for up to 80 hours and results from the excessive stimulation of pancreatic insulin by the drug. Glucose infusion is the treatment of choice but, since hyperglycaemia is also a potent stimulus to insulin release, hypoglycaemia may be poorly responsive to even high concentrations of infused glucose.

The somatostatin analogue octreotide (Sandostatin) has been used successfully to treat sulphonylurea-induced hypoglycaemia. It works by directly inhibiting the secretion of insulin from the islets of Langerhans. It can be given by subcutaneous injection three times daily or by continuous intravenous infusion.

References

1 Pramming S, Thorsteinsson B, Bendtson I, Binder C. Symptomatic hypoglycaemia in 411 Type-1 diabetic patients. *Diabetic Med* 1991;**8**: 217–22.

2 Gale EAM. The Somogyi effect. In: Nattrass M, ed. *Recent advances in diabetes 2*. Edinburgh: Churchill Livingstone, 1986:109–18.

3 Potter J, Clarke P, Gale EA *et al*. Insulin-induced hypoglycaemia in an accident and emergency department: the tip of an iceberg? *Br Med J* 1982;**285**:1180–2.

4 Diabetes Control and Complications Trial Research Group. The effect of intensive treatment of diabetes on the development and progression of long-term complications in insulin-dependent diabetes mellitus. *New Engl J Med* 1993;**329**:977–86.

5 UK Prospective Diabetes Study 16. Overview of 6 years therapy of Type II diabetes: a progressive disease. *Diabetologia* 1995;**44**:1249–58.

6 Jennings AM, Wilson RM, Ward JD. Symptomatic hypoglycaemia in NIDDM patients treated with oral hypoglycaemic agents. *Diabetes Care* 1989;**12**:203–8.

7 Macdonald MJ. Post-exercise late-onset hypoglycaemia in insulin-dependent diabetic patients. *Diabetes Care* 1987;**10**:584–8.

8 Fanelli CG, Epifano L, Rambotti AM *et al*. Meticulous prevention of hypoglycaemia normalises the glycaemic thresholds and magnitude of most neuroendocrine responses to, symptoms of, and cognitive function during hypoglycaemia in intensively treated Type-1 patients with short term IDDM. *Diabetes* 1993;**42**:1683–9.

9 Bolli G, De Feo P, Compagnucci P *et al*. Abnormal glucose counter-regulation in insulin-dependent diabetes mellitus. Interaction of anti-insulin antibodies and impaired glucagon and epinephrine secretion. *Diabetes* 1983;**32**:134–41.

10 Asplund K, Wiholm B-E, Lithner F. Glibenclamide-associated hypoglycaemia—a report of 57 cases. *Diabetologia* 1983;**24**:412.

11 Collier A, Steedman DJ, Partick AW *et al*. Comparison of intravenous glucagon and dextrose in the treatment of severe hypoglycaemia in an Accident and Emergency Department. *Diabetes Care* 1987;**10**:712–15.

12 Tunbridge WMG. Factors contributing to the deaths of diabetics under fifty years of age. *Lancet* 1981;**i**:569–72.

5 Diabetes and surgery

GEORGE HALL

Diabetes is the commonest endocrine problem in surgical patients: it is essential that all staff, who look after patients in the perioperative period, understand the disease, its complications, and management. Fortunately, the topic is reviewed regularly in the anaesthetic and surgical literature.[1,2] Diabetic patients usually present for surgery because of complications of the disease, for example cataract extraction, vascular surgery, coronary artery surgery, and renal transplantation. Byyny estimated that a diabetic patient had a 50% likelihood of needing surgery for a related complication.[3] With improvements in care, this is probably an underestimate in the late 1990s. The greater frequency of diabetic patients presenting for major surgery, such as coronary artery bypass grafting and renal transplantation, is a striking feature of modern surgical practice. For example, in one major cardiac unit the number of diabetic patients undergoing coronary artery bypass grafting increased from 4% in 1984 to 13% in 1990, and is expected to exceed 20% by the end of the decade. Amputation of a gangrenous leg is a common procedure and it is interesting to note the decline in mortality since the introduction of insulin and then antibiotics. In the 1930s mortality after this operation was about 50% and was still >20% in the 1950s. With the widespread availability of good diabetic and microbiological management, the mortality in the 1970s remained around 10%. Indeed, local audit data in busy vascular units indicates that amputation in the late 1990s is still associated with a mortality rate of 5–10%.

Surgical risk

Many early studies concluded that diabetic patients were at greater risk of postoperative morbidity, and even mortality, than

102

non-diabetic patients for a variety of major surgical procedures. However, more recent work has shown that, if they are carefully matched with an appropriate control group, there is no increased risk.[4] Unfortunately, much of this information has been determined retrospectively, and there is a need for a large, prospective study. There is considerable evidence, however, that diabetic patients undergoing cardiac surgery have increased in-hospital mortality that exceeds control patients by at least 50%.[2,5] The reasons for this are unknown, but are probably similar to those considered responsible for the excess mortality in diabetic patients with myocardial infarction (Chapter 7). If so, then intensive metabolic control in the perioperative period may improve outcome.

The determination of preoperative characteristics that would identify diabetic patients at increased risk in general surgery has been studied by MacKenzie and Charlson.[6] It was notable that diabetes itself was the critical variable, not whether it was type 1 or type 2 diabetes, nor the preoperative glucose concentration. The predictors of non-cardiac complications (11%) were the presence of microvascular complications (neuropathy, retinopathy, nephropathy), peripheral vascular disease with infection, and congestive cardiac failure or valve disease. Cardiac complications (7%) were predicted by age >75 years, and the presence of congestive cardiac failure or valve disease. Postoperative mortality was predicted only by congestive cardiac failure or valve disease, an expected finding as heart failure indicates a poor prognosis in many scoring systems for assessing surgical risk. The practical corollary is that diabetic patients with cardiac failure should only be operated on for emergency procedures, and their management must be undertaken by senior staff. If at all possible, cardiac failure should be controlled first.

Aims of management

The aims of metabolic management of the diabetic patient in the perioperative period are:

- Avoid hypoglycaemia.
- Avoid *excessive* hyperglycaemia.
- Prevent protein catabolism and lipolysis.
- Avoid electrolyte disorders (particularly loss of potassium, magnesium, and phosphate).

103

Avoiding hypoglycaemia is particularly important during anaesthesia. It is often said that it cannot be detected under general anaesthesia, but autonomic signs, such as tachycardia and sweating, may be seen (Chapter 4), although there are many other causes of these physiological changes during surgery and anaesthesia. Nevertheless, because of this fear of undetected hypoglycaemia, anaesthetists and surgeons have opted for "safe", i.e. high, glucose values. The ideal upper limit for blood glucose concentrations in the perioperative period is a contentious subject. It is noticeable, however, that the upper limit has declined steadily in the past 30 years. Many authorities now recommend that blood glucose values should be kept below 12 mmol/litre. This view is due, in part, to the accumulating evidence that shows deleterious effects of glucose concentrations >14 mmol/litre on a variety of biological functions necessary for wound healing and repair. Furthermore, ischaemic damage to the central nervous system and myocardium is exacerbated at a similar concentration, as a consequence of severe, prolonged lactic acidosis. Although this phenomenon is well recognised in neurosurgical units, where it is often difficult to find 5% glucose solution for intravenous infusion, it appears to be less understood in cardiac surgical units.

The experimental basis for impaired wound healing at high glucose concentrations is excellent, but the clinical effects are less evident. However, a recent study of over 4000 patients, who had undergone coronary artery bypass grafting, found that, if on admission to the ITU the blood glucose value was >11.1 mmol/litre, then the incidence of surgical infection was 4.5 times greater than if the circulating value was <11.1 mmol/litre. This finding, applied to diabetic and non-diabetic patients, strongly suggested that infection resulted solely from hyperglycaemia.

Metabolic problems with surgery

The metabolic management of the diabetic patient in the perioperative period, the maintenance of stable blood glucose values, and prevention of excessive lipolysis, protein catabolism and electrolyte loss, is hindered by several, inevitable, physiological factors:

- starvation
  - preoperative
  - postoperative

- hormonal and metabolic response to surgery
- immobilisation.

The need for prolonged starvation before elective surgery has been challenged recently, and in many hospitals food is allowed until four hours before surgery, and clear fluids until two hours before operation. This change from the old adage "starve from midnight" is particularly beneficial for the diabetic patient. Nevertheless, the possibility of gastroparesis, with delayed stomach emptying in the diabetic patient with autonomic neuropathy, must be considered. Postoperative starvation, either voluntary or enforced, is less easy to combat, and is particularly bad for metabolic control. Prophylaxis against nausea and vomiting should be considered, and these unpleasant sequelae treated vigorously if they occur.

The endocrine and metabolic response to surgery has been investigated in detail[7] in non-diabetic people, and its size is roughly proportional to the severity of the surgery. Diabetic patients with an absolute (type 1) or relative (type 2) deficiency of insulin are less able to respond to the catabolic stress of surgery, and unless this is taken into account, significant hyperglycaemia can develop in the perioperative period. For example, cataract extraction results in a short-lived rise in blood glucose (about four hours), whereas cardiac surgery evokes metabolic changes that can last for several days. The endocrine response can be summarised as enhanced catabolic and impaired anabolic hormone secretion. Increased release of catecholamines, cortisol, and growth hormone stimulates glycogenolysis and gluconeogenesis, and inhibits uptake of glucose peripherally. These changes in glucose metabolism are worsened by the failure of insulin secretion to respond to the increased blood glucose in the immediate perioperative period. This is thought to be mediated by the inhibitory alpha-adrenergic effects of circulating catecholamines on the beta-cells of the pancreas. Later in the perioperative period, insulin secretion recovers, but the biochemical effects of the hormone are impaired—the phase of "insulin resistance". Thus, surgery is associated with an absolute, or relative, deficiency of insulin.

These hormonal changes also affect protein metabolism. In minor and intermediate surgery, protein anabolism is inhibited, but in major surgery both suppression of synthesis and increased muscle protein breakdown occur. Lipid metabolism has received little attention, perhaps because surprisingly few changes occur except for increased lipolysis and ketogenesis once postoperative starvation is well established. It must be emphasised that these changes are found in non-diabetic patients and make metabolic control in diabetics even more difficult.

Postoperative immobilisation also contributes to glucose intolerance and depresses muscle protein synthesis. Early ambulation after surgery is encouraged for a variety of reasons, such as the prevention of deep vein thrombosis, and it also aids metabolic homeostasis. The importance of adequate postoperative analgesia is that it should permit rapid mobilisation.

Preoperative evaluation

At one time textbooks recommended that all diabetic patients should be admitted to hospital 48–72 hours before surgery so that their diabetic control could be assessed and changes made, if required. In a busy hospital, there may have been little time to evaluate a patient with diabetes before major surgery. In the absence of full patient notes, the following basic evaluation is essential in all diabetic patients (Box 5.1).

Thus, the basic evaluation consists of a simple history and examination, particularly of the cardiovascular system. The important tests are:

- blood glucose (fasting and post-prandial)
- urinalysis (ketones and protein)
- blood urea, creatinine and electrolytes
- haemoglobin
- ECG.

Other investigations may be necessary if indicated clinically

Tests for the presence of diabetic autonomic neuropathy (DAN) are not routine, but its presence may be indicated by symptoms such as postural hypotension, gastric atony, diarrhoea, sweating, impotence, and urinary problems. An increased resting heart rate indicates parasympathetic abnormalities and the Q–T interval may be prolonged. A useful indicator of the likelihood of the presence of DAN is hypertension. In the absence of hypertension it has been shown that the incidence of DAN is low (<10%).[8]

Box 5.1 Information needed in diabetic patients

Essential information
- Diabetes
  - type 1 or type 2, duration
- Drugs
  - current therapy (allergies)
- Cardiovascular disease
  - hypertension
  - ischaemic heart disease (ECG)
  - peripheral vascular disease
  - congestive cardiac failure
  - valve disease
  - haemoglobin
- Renal disease
  - blood urea, creatinine and electrolytes
  - urinary protein
- Metabolic control
  - blood glucose (fasting and post-prandial)
  - urinary ketones
- Neuropathy
  - sensory
- Eyes
  - proliferative retinopathy
- Musculoskeletal
  - stiff joint syndrome (SJS) (positive prayer sign)

Additional evaluation
Other useful factors in evaluating the diabetic patient before surgery include:

- Metabolic control
  - glycosylated haemoglobin (fructosamine)
- Neuropathy
  - autonomic
- Respiratory function
  - FEV_1 and FVC.

The importance of DAN is the resulting gastroparesis with an increased risk of regurgitation and aspiration on induction of anaesthesia. Cardiovascular lability is increased in the perioperative period with more vasopressor drugs needed to ensure cardiovascular stability.[9] It is possible that DAN was responsible for the occasional, unexplained cardiac arrests found immediately after surgery.

The stiff-joint-syndrome (SJS) or diabetic cheiroarthropathy is particularly important to anaesthetists as it indicates that there is an increased likelihood of difficult endotracheal intubation. First described by Salzarulo and Taylor,[10] it is usually found in type 1 diabetes patients with a rapidly progressive microangiopathy, short stature, tight waxy skin and limited joint mobility. The presence of a "positive prayer sign" is indicative of the SJS; patients are unable to approximate the palmer surface of the phalangeal joints. Neck mobility is impaired with particularly limited extension at the atlantoaxial joint. The incidence of SJS is reported at around 30% in type 1 diabetes patients.

If proliferative retinopathy is present, marked increases in arterial pressure must not occur, as they greatly increase the risk of vitreous haemorrhage. It is important to block the hypertensive response to laryngoscopy and intubation, extubation, as well as surgical trauma and severe pain postoperatively.

Metabolic management

Many ways of managing the diabetic patient during and after surgery have been described. There is no universally accepted method and this probably reflects the lack of adequately controlled studies with large numbers of patients. Furthermore, several different end-points have been used, such as control of blood glucose, duration of hospital stay and even morbidity.

A simple approach, agreed and understood by all medical and nursing staff, is the first essential requirement. A local protocol is particularly helpful. It is not uncommon for the diabetic management to be started by physicians, undertaken on the day of surgery by anaesthetists, and left to surgical staff for the rest of the hospital stay. Not surprisingly, major problems sometimes occur. The following recommendations have been found to work safely and reliably in busy hospital practice and refer to diabetic patients who require surgery as inpatients.

Type 1 diabetes

All patients undergoing surgery must be treated with an intra-venous glucose–insulin–potassium (GIK) regimen. Subcutaneous insulin is not used because of the increased variability in absorption which results from marked fluctuations in subcutaneous blood flow in the perioperative period.[11] A normal diet and the usual dose of insulin are taken on the day before surgery. If possible, diabetic patients are put first on morning operating lists. This minimises the duration of starvation and ensures that full laboratory facilities and expert help are available postoperatively, if required. As patients are starved from early morning, breakfast is omitted, and a GIK infusion started. If the patient is scheduled for an afternoon operating list, a light breakfast is eaten and half the usual morning dose of short-acting insulin given. The GIK regimen is started at midday. Intravenous insulin is continued until after the patient has resumed eating. The first meal in the postoperative period is preceded by s.c. insulin, and i.v. infusion is maintained for two hours after food. Frequent estimation of blood glucose values is essential.

There are two main methods of administering i.v. insulin:

- Alberti regimen
- sliding scale regimen.

Alberti regimen

This was described 20 years ago[12] and consists of the following mixture which is usually appropriate to maintain blood glucose values of 6–12 mmol/litre:

500 ml 10% glucose solution
15 units soluble insulin
10 mmol potassium

The usual infusion rate is 100 ml/h, and the amounts of insulin and potassium are changed depending on the blood glucose and plasma potassium concentrations. The major advantage of the Alberti regimen is safety. If the i.v. infusion is stopped inadvertently, or if the patient suddenly receives the complete bag of 10% glucose in a few minutes, there is no risk of obtaining substrate without insulin, or vice versa. The major disadvantage is its inflexibility. If the insulin or potassium content has to be changed, the bag has to be thrown away and a new one mixed. This can cause problems on some wards with nursing staff unwilling to take the responsibility of adding insulin to a solution for intravenous use. With the increased safety and reliability of syringe pumps, attention has moved from the Alberti regimen to the sliding scale regimen.

Sliding scale regimen

Two separate infusions are used, mixed just before the intravenous cannula, with a non-return valve to ensure that only the mixture enters the circulation if the cannula is flushed:

10% glucose solution with 10 or 20 mmol potassium chloride soluble insulin solution of 1 unit/ml (syringe pump).

The insulin solution is prepared by diluting 50 units of soluble insulin in 50 ml 0.9% saline solution. The infusion rate of glucose is again 100 ml/h, and the rate of insulin infusion is varied to maintain an appropriate blood glucose concentration. This regimen has improved flexibility compared with the Alberti technique, because only the glucose solution is changed if the potassium input has to be altered. The amount of insulin adsorbed to the syringe and tubing from this concentrated solution is small, so that, for practical purposes, the infusion rate is equal to the rate at which insulin is given: 3 ml/h $\equiv$ 3 units insulin/h. The sliding scale regimen does *not* have the inherent safety of the Alberti regimen and vigilance is essential. Three typical sliding scale regimens are shown in Table 5.1. Scale 1 is often appropriate for stable patients with a daily insulin requirement of <30 units, scale 2 is useful in patients with daily insulin requirements of 30–60 units, and scale 3 in those patients who usually need >60 units of insulin per day, or are unstable with an intercurrent illness.

Practical points of management (Figure 5.1)

There are several, important, practical points of management of patients receiving a GIK infusion.

Table 5.1   Typical sliding scale regimens in type 1 diabetes

Bl. glucose (mmol/litre)	Insulin infusion (units/h)		
	Scale 1	Scale 2	Scale 3
<3.9	0	0	0
4.0–6.9	0.25	0.5	0.5
7.0–9.9	0.5	1	2
10.0–14.9	1	2	3
15.0–19.9	2	3	4
>20.0	3	4	6

- The Alberti regimen assumes that the insulin requirements are 0.3–0.4 units/g glucose. This is increased in the following medical conditions:
  - liver disease
  - obesity
  - severe infections
  - concurrent steroid therapy.
- Patients with modest insulin requirements ($\leqslant 30$ units insulin/day) will often need only about 50 units of insulin (one syringe) in the first 24 hours after surgery. This avoids the need to prepare another syringe in the night.
- The initial rate of insulin infusion with the sliding scale regimen can be derived approximately as follows:

$$\frac{\text{blood glucose (mmol/litre)}}{5} = \text{units insulin/hour}$$

- The key to successful management is to measure blood glucose values frequently and take appropriate action. During cardiac surgery it may be necessary to measure blood glucose as often as every 20–30 min, but hourly or two hourly intervals are usual in routine orthopaedic surgery.
- Modern bedside methods of glucose estimation are easy, rapid, and usually accurate, provided they are used correctly. It is important, however, to check the accuracy of meters by occasionally sending concurrent blood samples to the main laboratory.
- The "ideal range" of blood glucose concentrations is difficult to define, but 6–12 mmol/litre would be a reasonable target to aim for.
- Serum potassium needs to be measured less often; we suggest at alternate glucose estimations. The ideal range is 4.0–5.0 mmol/litre, but extra care is necessary if renal impairment is present.
- There is no simple measure of lipolysis and ketogenesis in the perioperative period other than urinary ketones, and there are often practical difficulties in obtaining a urine specimen. In major surgery, with access to arterial samples, blood gas analysis and calculation of the standard bicarbonate and base deficit indicates the presence and severity of a metabolic acidosis. If circulating lactate values can also be measured, then any residual acidosis is likely to reflect ketoacidosis.

111

Ward		Enter details or affix patient sticker	
Date of surgery		Surname	
Surgeon		Forename	
Anaesthetist		Age/DoB	
Physician		Sex	

Planned surgical procedure	

Diabetic history		Complications	Tick if yes
Date of diagnosis	Date insulin started	Hypertension	
		Ischaemic heart disease	
Usual insulin dose	Usual diabetic tablets	Peripheral vascular disease	
		Peripheral neuropathy	
		Retinopathy	
		Proteinuria	
		Raised creatinine	
		Autonomic neuropathy	
Pre-op blood glucose	mmol/litre	time	
		AT RISK FEET	YES/NO

Anaesthetist to indicate which regimen is required when patient goes to theatre			
Dual infusion regimen • 50 units soluble insulin in 50ml 0.9% saline in syringe pump • 500ml 10% dextrose plus 1g KCl (according to table below)		*GKI regimen* • 500ml dextrose plus 1g KCl • x units of insulin (see below) (according to table below)	
Pre-op blood glucose mmol/litre	Insulin rate	Pre-op blood glucose mmol/litre	X U of insulin to add to bag
0.0–3.9	0	0.0–3.9	3
4.0–6.9	0.5	4.0–6.9	6
7.0–9.9	1	7.0–9.9	9
10.0–14.9	2	10.0–14.9	12
15.0–19.9	3	15.0–19.9	15
20+	4	20+	20

Dextrose infusion at 100ml/h. Check blood glucose hourly and change insulin accordingly.

IMMEDIATE POSTOPERATIVE MANAGEMENT	
Medical/surgical team	Anaesthetist

Figure 5.1   Management of diabetes during surgery. Patient record form.

Type 2 diabetes

Williams has drawn attention to a common misconception amongst some doctors that type 2 diabetes is "mild", is easy to treat and that tight metabolic control is unnecessary.[13] He states that only blood glucose values <10 mmol/litre are acceptable, even after meals. It could be argued that similar tight control is merited in the perioperative period.

There is considerable disagreement amongst clinicians about how these patients requiring surgery as inpatients should be managed. The simple approach is to give insulin to all patients either by the Alberti regimen or sliding scale regimen as described above. This is essential for major surgery, cardiac surgery, vascular surgery, or intra-abdominal surgery, regardless of whether treatment is by diet alone, or diet and oral hypoglycaemic drugs.

However, there is some evidence that for moderate and minor surgery, such as transurethral resection of the prostate, the use of a GIK regimen increases the incidence of metabolic abnormalities.[14] In these circumstances, it is usual to simply omit the oral hypoglycaemic drug(s) on the day of surgery and only start a GIK infusion if blood glucose control is difficult. As in type 1 diabetes patients, it is essential to measure blood glucose concentrations frequently and take appropriate action. Type 2 diabetes patients must be treated just as carefully as type 1 patients.

- Occasionally, oral hypoglycaemic drugs are given on the morning of surgery, in error. This usually happens with cardiac and vascular surgical patients, as the nursing staff are aware of the importance of maintaining therapy with cardioactive drugs in the perioperative period. More frequent blood glucose estimations are then needed, particularly after surgery. Occasionally glucose infusions are necessary in patients undergoing minor surgery.
- Chlorpropamide and glibenclamide are associated with an increased risk of hypoglycaemia (see Chapter 4) and may cause problems in surgery and postoperatively. The former drug has a long half-life (>30 h) which is prolonged further by renal impairment. Glibenclamide and its active metabolites accumulate within the beta-cells of the pancreas.
- Patients who are usually well controlled, but present on the evening before surgery with unsatisfactory blood glucose values (>15 mmol/litre), should be given 10 units of isophane insulin

subcutaneously. A GIK regimen is usually required on the day of surgery.

- Patients who are managed successfully without a GIK regimen for intermediate and minor surgery may need occasional s.c. insulin postoperatively to control the hyperglycaemia.

Anaesthetic considerations

There is no evidence that the anaesthetic technique affects morbidity and mortality in diabetic patients. Local anaesthetic techniques with an awake patient are often favoured as they can decrease the catabolic hormonal response to surgery and so improve metabolic control,[15] and also allow the onset of hypoglycaemia to be recognised. Furthermore, there is usually less postoperative nausea and vomiting and the patients resume normal eating and drinking earlier than with general anaesthesia. For example, spinal analgesia is often used for amputation of the foot or leg, and peribulbar blockade provides excellent operating conditions for cataract extraction. There are considerable data *in vitro* to show that all volatile anaesthetic agents inhibit glucose-stimulated insulin secretion. At present, there is little clinical evidence to support these observations, but it is possible that volatile agents may be contraindicated in type 2 diabetes patients.

It is often stated that lactate-containing solutions must not be infused i.v. in diabetic patients, because the lactate load undergoes gluconeogenesis and greatly exacerbates the hyperglycaemia.[16] The evidence to support this view is sparse and many anaesthetists infuse one or two litres of Hartmann's solution (lactate 29 mmol/litre) routinely during surgery. An important consideration in the choice of i.v. fluids is that the use of only a GIK infusion often results in marked hyponatraemia postoperatively (plasma Na^+ 120–130 mmol/litre). Therefore, any additional requirement for crystalloids is best met by the administration of sodium chloride 0.9% solution. (Note that most colloids, gelatins and etherified starch solutions are dissolved in sodium chloride 0.9% solution.)

Packs of red cell concentrates contain glucose and lactate (substrate and metabolite respectively), so that the rapid infusion of only a few packs may be associated with a sudden increase in blood glucose concentration. Obviously, if blood transfusion is required, nothing can be done about this additional glucose load.

Adequate analgesia after surgery is essential in diabeti
because good pain relief decreases catabolic hormone
Non-steroidal anti-inflammatory drugs must be used witl
if renal impairment is present, or suspected, particularl
elderly, because of the risk of precipitating a deterioration in renal
function or gastrointestinal haemorrhage. Postoperative nausea and
vomiting should be prevented, if possible, and otherwise treated
aggressively. The diabetic patient needs to resume oral intake as
soon as possible.

Postoperative care

The metabolic and endocrine response to surgery continues into
the postoperative period and can last for several days (see above).
It is notable that many catabolic hormonal responses are maximal,
not during surgery but on return to the ward. Additional factors
that contribute to catabolism postoperatively include hypoxaemia,
hypotension, infection, and immobilisation. Loss of appetite is an
almost inevitable consequence of major surgery.

It is logical, therefore, to continue the same standard of care that
was provided for the patient during surgery into the postoperative
period. However, the practical implementation of this policy is
difficult. There is often no guidance on who will manage the
diabetic patient in these circumstances, so that it becomes the
problem of a preregistration surgical house officer. The instructions
given by the anaesthetist for the control of blood glucose may
be used in the early postoperative period. Further anaesthetic
involvement is difficult because of continuing theatre commitments.

Postoperative glucose control is best achieved with an intravenous
insulin sliding scale and a glucose/potassium infusion. Insulin
infusion rates are adjusted according to bedside capillary glucose
results, usually done every 1–4 hours, depending on how stable
the patient is. This method has the added advantage of allowing
an estimate of daily insulin requirements that can be helpful when
transferring the patient back to subcutaneous insulin (Chapter 2).

Obviously, maintenance of adequate oxygenation and blood
pressure is important in all patients following surgery, but it is of
even greater significance in diabetic patients who frequently have
associated cardiac and renal dysfunction. Intravenous fluid
administration must be monitored carefully to ensure appropriate
cardiac filling and renal perfusion. Although urine output is

commonly used as an indicator of the adequacy of the circulating blood volume, it must be remembered that glycosuria will induce an osmotic diuresis.

Special situations

Day-case surgery

When day-case surgery was introduced, diabetes was considered a medical contraindication. Economic factors soon dictated that stable diabetic patients underwent surgery and were discharged on the same day. Common procedures carried out as day-cases are shown in Box 5.2.

Box 5.2 Day-case surgery

- *General surgical*
  - hernia repair
  - varicose veins
  - removal of hydrocele
  - circumcision
  - vasectomy
  - removal of skin lesions
- *Orthopaedic*
  - arthroscopy
  - carpal tunnel release
- *Chronic pain management*
  - nerve blocks

- *ENT*
  - submucous resection of nasal septum
  - sinus washouts
  - nasal polypectomies
- *Maxillofacial*
  - wisdom teeth
  - apicectomies
- *Gynaecology*
  - laparoscopy
  - sterilisation
  - dye insufflation
  - hysteroscopies

With careful selection, major problems are uncommon but there is little information at present on overall safety and metabolic control in subsequent days. An important variable in selecting patients with diabetes for day surgery is their home situation, together with a judgement of how well they understand and manage their diabetes.

For type 1 diabetes patients, half the normal dose of insulin is given in the morning; the patient is starved, operated on first and *must* be able to resume normal oral intake by lunchtime. Some anaesthetists favour the "no breakfast—no insulin" approach, but this may be associated with a greater risk of ketoacidosis. Rapid recovery of a pain-free patient without nausea and vomiting is essential. Additional soluble insulin may be needed to cover lunch, and the normal dose of insulin can usually be given with the evening meal.

Type 2 diabetes patients must also be stable metabolically. Any oral hypoglycaemic drugs are omitted, and it is usually only necessary to check the blood glucose on the morning of surgery and immediately after surgery.

Diabetes management plans should be agreed with the medical and nursing staff, and patient, and these must be simple, safe, and fully understood by all who use them. A summary of guidelines for management of patients undergoing same-day surgery is shown in Box 5.3 and Tables 5.2 and 5.3.

Box 5.3 General principles for day-case/ short-stay surgery

- *Aims*
  - avoid hypoglycaemia
  - avoid gross hyperglycaemia (>15 mmol/litre)
  - avoid ketoacidosis

- **All** patients should be listed *as early as possible* on the operating list

- *Starvation*

Morning list 08.30 start	Afternoon list 13.30 start
• no food from midnight	• light breakfast at 07.30
• free fluids if desired until 05.30	• free fluids if desired until 10.30
• then nil by mouth until return from theatre	• then nil by mouth until return from theatre

Diabetic patients should only be discharged home if they can eat and drink normally

---

Pregnancy

Women with type 1 diabetes become increasingly insulin resistant during the third trimester of pregnancy. To maintain optimal glycaemic control it is usually necessary to increase doses of insulin, often by as much as 100–200%, compared with prepregnancy doses. Both obstetric and diabetic considerations determine the mode of delivery, but in many hospitals up to 50% of women with

Table 5.2　Management of type 2 diabetes patients on diet or oral hypoglycaemics undergoing same-day surgery with local or general anaesthetic

Timing	Morning list	Afternoon list
Day before surgery	Normal diet $\pm$ tablets (If in hospital check capillary glucose at 22.00. Give 10 units isophane insulin if >15 mmol/litre)	Normal diet $\pm$ tablets
Day of surgery	No breakfast/omit tablets Capillary glucose prior to theatre If >15 mmol/litre start i.v. insulin sliding scale If <5 mmol/litre start 5% dextrose at 100 ml/h	Light breakfast/ usual tablets Capillary glucose at 12.00 am If >15 mmol/litre start i.v. insulin sliding scale If <5 mmol/litre start 5% dextrose at 100 ml/h
Postoperative care	Capillary glucose on return to ward Resume diet and tablets If >15 mmol/litre give 6 units soluble insulin and repeat after 2 hours	Capillary glucose on return to ward Resume diet and tablets If >15 mmol/litre give 6 units soluble insulin and repeat after 2 hours

Table 5.3　Management of type 1 or insulin-treated type 2 diabetes patients undergoing same-day surgery with local or general anaesthetic

Timing	Morning list	Afternoon list
Day before surgery	Normal diet and insulin	Normal diet and insulin
Day of surgery	Half normal morning insulin dose Capillary glucose every 2 hours If >15 mmol/litre start i.v. insulin sliding scale If <5 mmol/litre start 5% dextrose at 100 ml/h	Half normal morning insulin dose Capillary glucose every 2 hours If >15 mmol/litre start i.v. insulin sliding scale If <5 mmol/litre start 5% dextrose at 100 ml/h
Postoperative care	Capillary glucose on return to ward Give 6 units soluble insulin, s.c. if >15 mmol/litre and repeat glucose in 2 hours Resume normal diet and insulin at lunchtime or evening meal	Capillary glucose on return to ward Give 6 units soluble insulin, s.c. if >15 mmol/litre and repeat glucose in 2 hours Resume normal diet and insulin with evening meal

diabetes will be delivered by Caesarean section, in some cases as an emergency. Blood glucose management during labour should be sufficiently well controlled to allow emergency Caesarean section should this be necessary. Since women are usually kept on clear fluids once labour is established, it is simplest to use an insulin sliding scale regimen with hourly capillary blood glucose testing to control the metabolic state. The target blood glucose range should be 4–8 mmol/litre, which is lower than for surgery, partly because women in labour are conscious and therefore able to detect hypoglycaemia, and partly because higher maternal glucose levels cross the placenta and stimulate fetal insulin; this may increase the risk of neonatal hypoglycaemia. Similar considerations apply to the measurement of laboratory glucose and potassium, as have been described above.

Following a successful delivery of the placenta the "insulin resistant" stage evaporates immediately and, when subcutaneous insulin is restarted, doses approximating to those used before pregnancy and *not* those used in the third trimester must be used. This information can be surprisingly difficult to obtain from the patient or their medical notes, and it is useful to record the antenatal insulin regimen on the patient's antenatal cooperation card as a matter of routine. It is also important to discuss which insulin regimen the patient wishes to use in the postnatal period. Some women previously on twice daily insulin and who required three or four insulin injections during the pregnancy prefer to remain on a basal bolus regimen.

Women with gestational diabetes who need insulin during the third trimester should also be managed using a GIK regimen during labour. Postnatally, glucose tolerance usually returns to normal, and all insulin therapy should be stopped once the third stage of labour has been completed. Those on diet alone do not usually need insulin during labour, although blood glucose should be routinely monitored and a GIK regimen started if it increases over 7 mmol/litre. Glucose tolerance should be assessed using a 75 g OGTT (see page 1) at the six week postnatal check-up and, since there is a 50% chance that type 2 diabetes will develop over a 15-year follow-up, annual fasting blood glucose checks should be arranged with the general practitioner. Dietary advice directed at trying to maintain a normal weight, together with regular exercise, is the only effective way of delaying progression to type 2 diabetes.

Children

Children with type 1 diabetes present for surgery occasionally. They must be managed with a GIK infusion and may need more intensive monitoring than adults. The sliding scale regimen is particularly appropriate because of its flexibility. Hyponatraemia can be troublesome in children and 4% glucose + 0.18% saline solution is often used for i.v. infusion in place of 10% or 5% glucose.

However, children rapidly become ketotic, and it is preferable to use a more concentrated glucose solution to which is added ampoules of saline 0.9% solution. A typical final concentration of Na^+ in the i.v. infusion is 50 mmol/litre ($\equiv$ saline 0.3% solution). Careful control of the rate of i.v. administration is essential in small children to prevent fluid overload. Intravenous access may be difficult until the child has been anaesthetised.

Emergency surgery

Any diabetic patient, presenting for emergency surgery must be managed with a GIK regimen. It is important to remember that DKA may present as an acute abdomen (Chapter 3). If circulating blood glucose values are high and marked ketonuria is present, these metabolic and fluid balance problems must be controlled *before* surgery (see Chapter 3). The patient may require admission to an Intensive Care Unit or High Dependency Unit for suitable monitoring to be instituted, and surgery should be delayed as long as possible. If severe fluid deficits are known, or suspected, then intravascular monitoring (direct arterial pressure and central venous pressure) is mandatory. The urgent nature of many surgical conditions is often in the minds of surgical trainees, and senior consultation may be necessary.

References

1 Hirsch IB, McGill JB, Cryer DE, White PF. Perioperative management of surgical patients with diabetes mellitus. *Anesthesiology* 1991;**74**: 346–59.
2 Milaskiewicz RM, Hall GM. Diabetes and anaesthesia: the past decade. *Br J Anaesth* 1992;**68**:198–206.
3 Byyny RL. Management of diabetes during surgery. *Postgrad Med* 1980;**70**:191–201.
4 Hjortrup A, Sorenson C, Dyremose E, Hjortso NC, Kehlet H. Influence of diabetes mellitus on operative risk. *Br J Surg* 1985;**75**: 783–5.
5 Lawrie GM, Morris GC, Glaeser DH. Influence of diabetes mellitus on the results of bypass surgery. *J Am Med Ass* 1986;**256**: 2967–71.

6 Mackenzie CR, Charlson ME. Assessment of perioperative risk in patients with diabetes mellitus. *Surg Gynecol Obstet* 1988;**167**:293–9.

7 Hall GM. Endocrine and metabolic responses to surgery and anaesthesia. In: Nimmo WS, Rowbotham DJ, Smith G, eds. *Anaesthesia*, 2nd edn. Oxford: Blackwells, 1994:595–605.

8 Maser RE, Pfeifer MA, Dorman JS, Kuller LH, Becker DJ, Orchard TJ. Diabetic autonomic neuropathy and cardiovascular risk. Pittsburgh epidemiology of diabetes complications study III. *Arch Intern Med* 1990;**150**:1218–22.

9 Burgos LG, Ebert TJ, Assiddao C *et al.* Increased intraoperative cardiovascular morbidity in diabetics with autonomic neuropathy. *Anesthesiology* 1989;**70**:591–7.

10 Salzarulo HH, Taylor LA. Diabetic "Stiff Joint Syndrome" as a cause of difficult endotracheal intubation. *Anesthesiology* 1986;**64**:366–8.

11 Hjortrup A, Madsbad S, Andersen M *et al.* Effect of major surgery on absorption of NPH insulin injected s.c. *Br J Anaesth* 1990;**64**:741–2.

12 Alberti KGMM, Thomas DJB. The management of diabetes during surgery. *Br J Anaesth* 1979;**51**:693–710.

13 Williams G. Management of non-insulin-dependent diabetes mellitus. *Lancet* 1994;**343**:95–100.

14 Thompson J, Husband DJ, Thai AC, Alberti KGMM. Metabolic changes in non-insulin-dependent-diabetes undergoing minor surgery: effect of glucose insulin potassium infusion. *Br J Surg* 1986;**73**:301–4.

15 Barker JP, Robinson PN, Vafidis GC, Burrin JM, Sapsed-Byrne S, Hall GM. Metabolic control of non-insulin-dependent diabetic patients undergoing cataract surgery: comparison of local and general anaesthesia. *Br J Anaesth* 1995;**74**:500–5.

16 Thomas DJB, Alberti KGMM. Hyperglycaemic effects of Hartmann's solution during surgery in patients with maturity onset diabetes. *Br J Anaesth* 1978;**50**:185–7.

6 Diabetes and investigations

Several radiological and endoscopic procedures require patients to starve before the test. A barium enema needs 24-hour preparation with purgation and a low residue diet. Hydrogen breath tests, for the investigation of lactose intolerance or intestinal bacterial overgrowth, involve taking a significant glucose load by mouth. Radiological procedures using intravenous contrast can also cause problems, particularly in patients with diabetic nephropathy and in those taking metformin. This chapter discusses how to manage patients who require hospital investigations particularly regarding their glycaemic control.

Who could run into problems?

Problems with glucose control are most likely to occur in patients with type 1 diabetes and in those with type 2 taking tablets or insulin. Patients who control their diabetes with diet alone should be treated in the same way as non-diabetics. When you are organising investigations, there is no substitute for good communications, and it is important for the referring doctor to inform the X-ray or endoscopy department that a patient referred for investigation has diabetes *and* to include details of their treatment. This seems rather obvious, but a study from Liverpool showed that this information was omitted in half of the requests to their X-ray department. As a result patients received no advice about how to modify their treatment.[1]

The solution is to develop agreed protocols, in discussion with the local diabetes specialist and relevant departments, tailored to specific investigation so that patients receive appropriate and consistent advice on how to modify their treatment. Such protocols should include agreed "ideal times" for patients to have investigations, usually first on a morning list, to make management as straightforward as possible. The following sections suggest protocols covering common investigations which require preparation involving starvation, purgation, or fluid restriction.

Investigations requiring starvation

A list of common radiologic and endoscopic procedures which require a minimum of eight hours' starvation is shown in Box 6.1.

Box 6.1 Investigations which require a minimum of eight hours' starvation in preparation

- *Radiological procedures*
  - barium meal $\pm$ follow through
  - small bowel meal
  - ultrasound examination of the liver and gallbladder
  - CT scanning of abdomen
  - cardiac or peripheral vascular angiography
  - MR scanning of the liver and gallbladder

- *Endoscopic procedures*
  - oesophagogastroduodenoscopy (OGD)
  - oesophageal dilatation
  - endoscopic retrograde cholecystopancreatography (ERCP)

If the investigation is to be done in the morning, patients are usually asked to starve from midnight. For those with diabetes the simplest and safest strategy is to schedule the investigation **first** on a morning list. If this is possible the patient should follow the advice shown in Box 6.2.

The doctor requesting the procedure should advise patients about how to control their blood glucose before the investigation and, ideally, this should be confirmed in writing when the appointment is made by the X-ray department using agreed guidelines.

Investigations requiring purgation

Barium enema and colonoscopic studies require purgation together with a low residue diet for 24 hours, in order to clean the colon of faecal residue. This usually involves two doses of a laxative such as Picolax. The patient is advised to eat a low-residue diet

123

Box 6.2 Advice for diabetic patients who have to starve for an investigation

- Take your usual diet and tablets/insulin the day before
- Do not have anything to eat or drink on the morning of the test and **DO NOT** take your usual dose of tablets or insulin
- Bring your tablets/insulin to the hospital
- You will be able to have your tablets or insulin, and your breakfast, once the test has been completed

---

(Box 6.3) for 24 hours, and this may present problems in blood glucose management, particularly in those patients on sulphonylureas or insulin.

The doctor requesting the investigation should advise the patient about how to cope with bowel preparation (Box 6.4).

Younger patients with a good understanding of their diabetes should be able to manage at home, provided that they can monitor

---

Box 6.3 Advice for patient on morning list for low-residue diet in preparation for a barium enema

Day before the examination

Throughout the preparation drink regular amounts of water or clear fluids.

At least 1 glass of water should be drunk every hour.

Before breakfast:	Take 1 sachet of Picolax mixed with water (no later than 8 am)
Breakfast:	1 boiled egg; 1 slice dry white toast; tea/coffee, no milk
Lunch:	Small portion of chicken or fish; NO vegetables; plain jelly; tea/coffee, no milk
Two hours after lunch:	Take second sachet of Picolax
Dinner:	Clear soup, Bovril or Oxo, plain fruit-flavoured jelly; tea/coffee, no milk

Day of examination

Breakfast:	1 boiled egg; 1 slice dry white toast; tea/coffee, no milk

---

Box 6.4 Advice for diabetic patients for bowel preparation

- *Oral hypoglycaemics*
  - Take half the usual dose of tablet(s) on the day of the bowel preparation **and** before breakfast on the morning of the test.
  - Monitor your blood glucose every 3–4 hours during the day.
  - If you have a hypoglycaemic episode you can take sugar by mouth. This will not affect the bowel preparation.
- *Insulin*
  - Reduce the usual insulin doses by half on the day of the bowel preparation **and** before breakfast on the morning of the test.
  - Monitor your blood glucose every 3–4 hours during the day.
  - You may need to adjust your insulin dose according to the results.
  - If you have a hypoglycaemic episode you can take sugar by mouth. This will not affect the bowel preparation.

---

their blood glucose. It is also reassuring for patients to be provided with contact numbers of their local diabetes service for advice if they have problems.

Some patients, particularly the elderly and those living alone find bowel preparation an arduous undertaking. Elderly patients on long acting sulphonylureas deserve special mention because of the risk of hypoglycaemia. They usually require admission to have their diabetes monitored and to obtain adequate bowel preparation. It is the responsibility of the doctor requesting the test to judge whether a patient is likely to cope with the preparation.

If the investigation is arranged for an afternoon list, bowel preparation is similar. Patients are also allowed a "light lunch" on the day of the test. Half the usual dose of tablets or insulin should be taken the morning before, and the morning of, the investigation. If the patient is already in hospital, a glucose, insulin, and potassium infusion is an alternative approach. Once the investigation is completed patients can resume their normal diet and treatment regimen.

Investigations requiring fluid restriction

Preparation for intravenous pyelography (IVP) requires fluid restriction for eight hours so that renal anatomy can be visualised.

This may present problems in patients with diabetes, particularly those with nephropathy or taking diuretics. Intravenous contrast may also compromise renal function and, if possible, an alternative technique such as renal ultrasound should be used. If an IVP is essential, fluid restriction should be avoided and renal function checked before and after the investigation. Metformin should be stopped 48 hours before the test.

Preparation for pelvic ultrasound requires that the patient drinks liberally to make sure the bladder is full before the test. This does not usually present problems in diabetes.

Investigations requiring intravenous contrast

The following case illustrates the potential risk of investigations using i.v. contrast medium.

Case Study 16

A 45-year-old woman with a 30-year history of type 1 diabetes was admitted for assessment of dry gangrene of her right hallux. She had required extensive photocoagulation for severe retinopathy and had been registered blind three years previously. Peripheral neuropathy had been present for a number of years, although she had no past history of proteinuria and her serum creatinine was 100 µmol/litre on admission. In addition to her insulin she was taking frusemide 40 mg/day for dependent oedema.

There were no pulses present in the foot or popliteal fossa, and a bruit was heard over the femoral artery. Arteriography was requested and, in preparation, she was required to restrict food and fluids for six hours. Her diabetes was controlled with an i.v. insulin sliding scale.

The arteriogram was performed without event but the following morning her serum creatinine had risen to 170 µmol/litre. Over the next two days the serum creatinine continued to increase and peaked at 340 µmol/litre. Her frusemide was stopped and she was treated with intravenous fluids with careful documentation of fluid balance. The serum creatinine gradually returned to normal over the next three days.

Those at greatest risk of acute exacerbations of renal function include patients with established nephropathy or other pre-existing renal disease. Patients with type 1 appear to be at greater risk than those with type 2 diabetes.

Avoiding the risk of contrast-induced renal impairment is best achieved by using, where possible, alternative non-invasive investigations such as Duplex ultrasound scanning or MR angiography. If intravenous contrast is the only option, it is important to avoid dehydration during preparation for the test, and to use as low a dose of contrast as possible. Potentially nephrotoxic drugs such as non-steroidal anti-inflammatory agents should be stopped and renal function should be carefully monitored after the procedure.

Metformin and intravenous contrast medium

In accord with the use of the data sheet recommendation for metformin, the UK Royal College of Radiologists has recently recommended that, to avoid any risk of lactic acidosis, metformin should be stopped for 48 hours prior to radiological procedures using intravenous contrast medium. These recommendations have been adopted by radiology departments in the UK, even though the actual risk of precipitating lactic acidosis is extremely small. It is, therefore important to notify X-ray departments if a patient is taking metformin so that appropriate advice can be sent to the patient with the appointment.

Investigations requiring oral glucose loading

Glucose-hydrogen breath tests are outpatient procedures to investigate suspected lactose intolerance or bacterial overgrowth of the small intestine, as may occur in autonomic neuropathy in long-standing diabetes. Patients starve from 10.00 pm the previous evening and avoid starchy carbohydrate such as bread, pasta, or rice the previous day. Depending on the test, patients drink 100 g glucose solution (472 ml Lucozade–bacterial overgrowth) or 50 g lactose dissolved in hot water (lactose tolerance test). Breath hydrogen is measured at regular intervals over two hours, after which the patient can eat and drink normally.

Hyperglycaemia following the oral glucose load is the main concern. It is sensible to check the fasting blood glucose on arrival. A value of >15 mmol/litre suggests very poor diabetic control, and it would be unwise to proceed with the investigation because of the risk of precipitating marked hyperglycaemia. If the fasting glucose is satisfactory, the patient should be given their normal

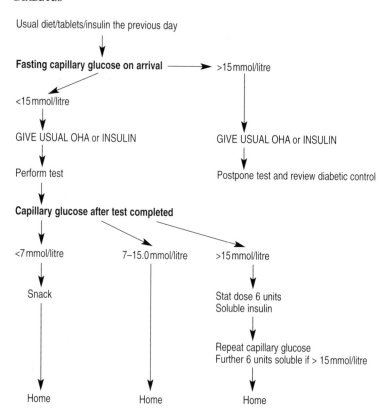

Usual diet/tablets/insulin the previous day

Fasting capillary glucose on arrival ⟶ >15 mmol/litre

<15 mmol/litre

GIVE USUAL OHA or INSULIN

Perform test

GIVE USUAL OHA or INSULIN

Postpone test and review diabetic control

Capillary glucose after test completed

<7 mmol/litre   7–15.0 mmol/litre   >15 mmol/litre

Snack

Stat dose 6 units
Soluble insulin

Repeat capillary glucose
Further 6 units soluble if > 15 mmol/litre

Home   Home   Home

Figure 6.1   Protocol for investigations requiring oral glucose loading.

tablets or insulin plus their oral glucose load. Once the test is completed, the glucose should be checked and, if unacceptably high, the patient should receive 6 units subcutaneous soluble insulin with repeat blood testing two hours later. This cycle can be repeated until the blood sugar has fallen to <15 mmol/litre. A suggested protocol is shown in Figure 6.1.

Reference

1 Eyre BE, Macfarlane IA, Reeve RG. Preparing diabetic patients for X-ray examination: potential hazards. *Br Med J* 1986;**292**:658.

7 Diabetes and ischaemic heart disease

Approximately 10% of patients admitted with acute myocardial infarction (AMI) have diabetes, and they are more likely to have longer and more complicated admissions. Both in-hospital and long-term mortality are approximately twice that of non-diabetic subjects with much of the excess mortality due to re-infarction or progressive heart failure. The diabetic patient with AMI is a "high-risk" patient in all respects. Readers who are interested in the underlying reasons for the excess cardiovascular risk in diabetes are referred to a recent extensive review.[1]

Hyperglycaemia is also important prognostically in patients with AMI who are not known to have diabetes. Of 248 non-diabetic patients admitted to a London teaching hospital, 49 (19.8%) had blood glucose concentrations >11 mmol/litre.[2] Their in-hospital mortality rate was 55% compared with 18% in the rest.

Recent clinical trials have provided evidence to guide clinical management of the diabetic patient with AMI and the secondary prevention of cardiovascular disease in those who survive. In this chapter, the presentation of AMI in diabetes will be reviewed. Management guidelines, with particular reference to controlling hyperglycaemia, the benefits and risks of thrombolysis, and secondary prevention of future vascular events will be described.

Presentation

The presentation of ischaemic heart disease is broadly similar to the non-diabetic population as in the following case history.

Case Study 17

A 57-year-old man with a seven-year history of type 2 diabetes was admitted with a three hour history of cardiac chest pain radiating to the neck and left arm and associated with sweating,

129

nausea, and vomiting. He was moderately overweight with a body mass index of 28.6 kg/m^2, and he smoked 10–15 cigarettes per day. He controlled his diabetes with diet and gliclazide (80 mg b.d.) and, at a recent clinic visit, his HBA$_{1c}$ was 7.8%. He had background retinopathy with macular involvement and had recently been put on the waiting list for laser photocoagulation.

On examination he was obviously in pain with a tachycardia, raised venous pressure, and bilateral basal crackles. There were no heart murmurs. An ECG showed acute ST elevation in the anterolateral leads, and an acute anterolateral myocardial infarction was diagnosed. Initial biochemistry showed a blood glucose of 15.4 mmol/litre, with a normal creatinine, and a serum potassium of 3.5 mmol/litre. A chest X-ray showed upper lobe blood diversion, Kerley B lines, and fluid in the horizontal fissure.

Whilst most patients have classical symptoms of ischaemic heart disease, some present with unusual or atypical features, such as episodic sweating or malaise, shortness of breath on exertion, or syncope. The development of congestive cardiac failure in a patient with diabetes may also be due to a painless AMI, where the onset may have been marked by "flu-like" symptoms or an episode of "indigestion" as shown in the following case.

Case Study 18

A 56-year-old lady with a six-year history of type 2 diabetes was referred to medical outpatients with a short history of progressive shortness of breath, orthopnoea, and paroxysmal nocturnal dyspnoea. She reported no severe chest pain but described a vague discomfort in the chest associated with malaise four weeks previously which she had put down to an "off day". Examination revealed a resting tachycardia, raised venous pressure, gallop rhythm, and bilateral basal crackles. Her ECG revealed a recent anterior Q-wave myocardial infarction, and the chest X-ray confirmed pulmonary oedema. An echocardiogram showed reduced anterior wall and septal motion with impaired left ventricular function. She was started on a combination of a loop diuretic and an ACE inhibitor with benefit, and aspirin was also started. Arrangements were made to check her fasting cholesterol and triglycerides.

A number of management issues are raised by the above cases. In the classical acute presentation, these revolve around the importance of glycaemic control and whether thrombolysis should be given. In both cases, secondary prevention of future vascular

---

Box 7.1 Key questions in managing AMI in diabetes

- What is the immediate and long-term prognosis?
- Is tight blood glucose control important and, if so, how should this be achieved?
- Should the patient receive thrombolysis?
- How can the risk of future AMI be minimised?

---

events is an important part of the management plan. The key questions relating to the management of AMI in diabetes are shown in Box 7.1.

What is the immediate and long-term prognosis?

Vascular disease is the major cause of death in diabetes, accounting for 40% of deaths in type 1 and up to 75% in type 2 diabetes. Most of these deaths are due to ischaemic heart disease with type 2 diabetes posing the greatest risk (Table 7.1).

Table 7.1   Causes of death in 448 patients with type 1 diabetes who died under 50 years of age[3] and 245 type 2 diabetes patients taking part in the UKPDS trial.[4]

Cause of death	Type 1 diabetes (%)	Type 2 diabetes (%)
Ischaemic heart disease	31	50
Cerebrovascular disease	7	7
Other vascular disease	3	N/A
Sudden	N/A	5
Renal failure	17	1
Ketoacidosis	16.5	0.5
Hypoglycaemia	4	0.5
Others	21.5	35

The statistics regarding AMI and diabetes are stark. Ischaemic heart disease is responsible for one in four diabetes-related hospital admissions, and such patients run a longer and more complicated hospital course (Table 7.2). Diabetes had a similar adverse effect on survival in both racial groups in the table. It can be seen from the Corpus Christi Heart Study data that the excess mortality is due mainly to "pump failure", even though infarct size was similar

131

Table 7.2   Data from the Corpus Christi Heart Study of Mexican-Americans and Non-Hispanic Whites, admitted with acute myocardial infarction between 1988–1990.[5]

Characteristic	Diabetic	Non-diabetic	P
Length of stay	12.1 days	8.9 days	<0.001
Peak creatinine kinase (MB fraction) (IU/litre)	757 ± 50	795 ± 46	0.59
Left ventricular ejection fraction (%)	53%	55%	0.03
Episodes of heart failure during admission	44.9%	25.2%	<0.05
Mortality			
28 days	10.1%	5.0%	<0.001
44 months	37.4%	23.3%	<0.001

between the two groups. The findings of the Corpus Christi study have been confirmed many times, and a number of possible explanations have been proposed:

- Patients with diabetes often have more severe and diffuse atheromatous coronary disease which may affect left ventricular function in AMI.
- Cardiac function may be affected as a result of pre-existing hypertension.
- Fibrosis occurs in the ventricular wall in patients with long-standing diabetes owing to microvascular tissue damage.[6]
- Autonomic neuropathy may impair the ability of the heart to cope with the haemodynamic changes.

The long-term prognosis following AMI is poor relative to non-diabetic subjects, mainly owing to an increased risk of heart failure.[7] The fact that one in three patients with diabetes who survive AMI are dead within three years emphasises the importance of effective secondary prevention in long-term management (see below).

Is blood glucose control important and, if so, how should this be achieved?

AMI generates a stress response with increased concentrations of several hormones including catecholamines and cortisol.[8] The magnitude of this response correlates with infarct size, left ventricular dysfunction, and, ultimately, prognosis. Hyperglycaemia is also related to the endocrine stress response of AMI and is itself an important prognostic marker with high blood glucose being associated with a worse prognosis. Whether this association is a direct adverse effect of hyperglycaemia or is related to the counterregulatory hormone response and, therefore, infarct size remains a source of debate.

The stress response to AMI also affects other metabolic pathways. Concentrations of free fatty acids increase in proportion to infarct size and, in animal models, these may cause arrhythmias and suppress cardiac contractility. Whether free fatty acids have adverse efects in AMI in man is unknown.

Insulin both controls hyperglycaemia and suppresses free fatty acid production, and is a logical way of controlling the metabolic changes associated with AMI. Low-dose sliding scale insulin regimens have been shown to be effective in controlling hyperglycaemia in AMI (Table 7.3).

Table 7.3 Protocol for the management of hyperglycaemia in patients presenting with AMI (adapted from Gwilt et al.)[9]

Capillary glucose (mmol/litre)	Insulin infusion rate (unit/h)
<4.0	0
4.0–8.0	1.0
8.1–12.0	2.0
>12.0	4.0

I.v. insulin sliding scale; 50 units *soluble* insulin in 50 ml 0.9% saline.
Hourly capillary glucose tests until <10 mmol/litre, then 2–4 hourly tests.

The important question of whether better metabolic control improves prognosis has been a subject of debate, with the few available studies providing conflicting evidence. Recently a large prospective randomised trial of insulin-glucose therapy in AMI from Scandinavia has provided evidence that intensive blood glucose control does improve prognosis. The DIGAMI (Diabetes Insulin Glucose Acute Myocardial Infarction)[10,11] investigators randomised 620 patients with AMI and an admission blood glucose >11 mmol/litre to receive either a 24-hour insulin infusion followed by intensive subcutaneous insulin therapy or to standard treatment. During three and a half years follow-up there were 102 deaths in the intensive treatment group and 138 in the control group, an 11% reduction in absolute mortality equivalent to one life saved for every nine patients treated.[11]

On the basis of the DIGAMI trial, the patient described in case study 17 is likely to benefit from an "intensive insulin" strategy with

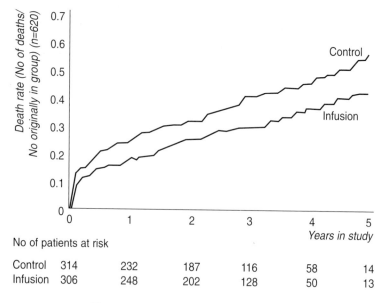

Figure 7.1   Survival benefit in DIGAMI trial.[11]

improved peri-infarct metabolic control, and then subcutaneous insulin to optimise diabetic control in the longer term. The protocol for acute control of hyperglycaemia in the DIGAMI study is shown in Box 7.2.[10]

The DIGAMI protocol is more complicated than a straight-forward sliding scale insulin regimen which many hospitals are familiar with. Since there are no published trials comparing the safety and effectiveness of different infusion regimens for control of hyperglycaemia in AMI, local facilities and experience should determine whether the DIGAMI protocol or a sliding scale regimen is used.

Potential problems

Day 1

There are two principal risks when an insulin infusion is given in the peri-infarct situation: hypoglycaemia and hypokalaemia. The risk of hypoglycaemia is partly related to the glycaemic targets which are set. In the feasibility study which preceded the DIGAMI trial, 28 episodes of hypoglycaemia (<3.0 mmol/litre) were recorded

Box 7.2 DIGAMI protocol for acute control of hyperglycaemia

Infusion mixture
500 ml of 5% dextrose with 80 units soluble insulin
Start with 30 ml/h
Check blood glucose after 1 hour
Adjust rate according to the protocol
Target blood glucose range 7–10.9 mmol/litre
Monitor blood glucose every 1–2 hours

Titrate infusion rate

Blood glucose (mmol/litre)	Adjustment
>15.0	Give 8 units soluble insulin as an i.v. bolus. Increase infusion rate by 6 ml/h
11.0–14.9	Increase infusion rate by 3 ml/h
7.0–10.9	Maintain current infusion rate
4.0–6.9	Decrease infusion rate by 6 ml/h
<4.0	Stop infusion until blood glucose is >7 mmol/litre. Give 20 ml of 30% glucose i.v. if symptomatic hypoglycaemia. Restart infusion with rate decreased by 6 ml/h

out of 158 patients treated, with a target blood glucose range of 7.0–10.9 mmol/litre, but the rate rose unacceptably with a target glucose range of 5.0–8.0 mmol/litre.

With an intravenous insulin infusion, there is a small risk of hypokalaemia, which is undesirable in the context of AMI. In the DIGAMI trial, serum potassium fell by 0.2 mmol/litre compared with 0.11 mmol/litre in the control group, although no patients had levels <3.5 mmol/litre. Serum potassium should be measured on admission and repeated 12 hours after starting insulin infusion. Appropriate oral or intravenous supplementation should be given to maintain the plasma potassium concentration >4.0 mmol/litre.

Day 2
The intensive treatment arm of the DIGAMI trial consisted of intravenous insulin-glucose infusion to control hyperglycaemia in the first 24 hours of admission followed by long-term, multidose subcutaneous insulin. It is not possible to determine whether the survival benefit in DIGAMI occurred as a result of improved

glucose control in the peri-infarct period, improved long-term diabetic control with insulin, or possibly withdrawal of oral hypoglycaemic drugs. This is particularly important because the greatest benefit was obtained in patients who were previously at low risk and not treated with insulin, such as described in case study 17 above. By no means all patients in this category will be able to cope with subcutaneous insulin therapy. In DIGAMI, 50% of patients were excluded because of an "inability or unwillingness to cope with injections", and it may be difficult in routine practice to identify these patients.

What should be advised? In practical terms the decision to recommend long-term subcutaneous insulin will have to be made on an individual basis, taking into account their general condition, preferences, and occupation. Discussion should include the pros and cons of insulin therapy; a demonstration injection may alleviate anxiety about coping with injections and allows patients to appreciate what is involved. The decision is probably best taken by an experienced diabetologist with support from a diabetes specialist nurse, who could then provide a full programme of education and support for those patients who agree to insulin therapy.

Should patients with diabetes receive thrombolysis?

Thrombolysis is an established treatment for patients with AMI and, in the International Study on Infarct Survival II (ISIS-II) trial,[12] was associated with a 20% reduction in overall mortality. It also works well in patients with diabetes, as can be seen in Table

Table 7.4 Annual in-hospital mortality for diabetic and non-diabetic patients admitted with confirmed acute myocardial infarction[13]

Year	Diabetic mortality (%)	Non-diabetic mortality (%)
1984	27.2	19.9
1985	22.0	21.3
1986	22.4	12.7
1987	30.5	16.5
1990	19.6	10.9 (Thrombolysis established)
1991	14.2	7.8
1992	15.7	6.4

7.4 which shows the effect on mortality, following its routine use in a CCU in Birmingham, UK.

In fact, diabetic subjects may benefit more than non-diabetics. The Fibrinolytic Trialists' Collaborative Group,[14] a meta-analysis of all thrombolytic trials of over 1000 patients, showed an absolute reduction in mortality of 3.7% in diabetics compared with 2.1% in non-diabetics, equivalent to four lives saved for every 100 patients treated, compared with two per 100 for non-diabetic subjects.

Despite this strong evidence of the benefit, several studies have shown that significantly fewer patients with diabetes receive thrombolysis compared with non-diabetic subjects. One explanation can be found in the data sheet for streptokinase which states that "caution is necessary in patients with diabetic retinopathy as there may be an increased risk of local bleeding". The belief that thrombolysis is contraindicated if a patient has retinopathy is widespread; a survey of junior hospital doctors in Scotland in 1994 showed that 80% believed retinopathy to be an absolute contraindication to thrombolysis.[15] In fact, the risk of intraocular haemorrhage with thrombolysis is extremely small: for example, in the GUSTO thrombolytic trial, no episodes of retinal haemorrhage were recorded in over 6000 treated diabetic patients.[16] There are also important issues concerning practical aspects of eye examination in coronary care, because of the pupillary constriction associated with opiate analgesia, which makes reliable retinal assessment almost impossible. Given the benefits of thrombolysis in subjects with diabetes it is not justified to withhold treatment, even in those patients with proliferative change (Box 7.3).

Box 7.3 Recommended thrombolysis

- A standard regimen of 1.5 million units of streptokinase should be infused over 1 hour as soon as possible after admission to a coronary care unit.
- Diabetic retinopathy is *not* a contraindication to thrombolysis. Do not delay thrombolysis while waiting for mydriatic drops to take effect.

The only exception may be the (rare) situation of a patient with a recent vitreous or preretinal haemorrhage. In this circumstance the risks of ocular complications will be greatest although vitreo-

137

retinal surgery now offers the prospect of restoration of sight even in the presence of extensive vitreous haemorrhage. Clinical judgement, together with, if possible, discussion of the options with the patient, would be needed for a decision to start thrombolysis.

Aspirin

The Antiplatelet Trialists' Collaboration reported 17% fewer vascular events in diabetic patients taking antiplatelet drugs compared with 22% reduction in non-diabetics (35 events prevented for every 1000 treated with diabetes).[17] There was a two-fold increase in the risk of cerebral haemorrhage, but the benefits of antiplatelet treatment outweigh this risk in patients with established coronary or cerebrovascular disease. Aspirin worked as well as other antiplatelet drugs, although there is some evidence to suggest that doses of 300 mg/day may be needed in diabetes because of increased platelet turnover.

Aspirin (300 mg o.d.) should be given to patients with diabetes admitted with AMI or unstable angina unless there are contraindications.

Management of AMI in diabetes—the first 24 hours

Patients with diabetes who present with suspected AMI are at high risk of complications, and should be managed on a coronary care unit with full defibrillation facilities. Ischaemic cardiac pain should be managed with diamorphine. They should receive aspirin on arrival, if this has not already been given on the way. If ECG criteria for thrombolysis are present, then 1.5 million units of streptokinase should be infused with appropriate monitoring. All patients with an admission glucose >11 mmol/litre should receive an intravenous insulin infusion as soon as possible (see above). Regular review is important with particular attention paid to clinical or radiological signs of heart failure, which may require stat doses of loop diuretic or intravenous infusion of a nitrate. The 4th International Study on Infarct Survival (ISIS-4) confirmed the safety of nitrates in almost 60 000 patients with suspected AMI, although no survival benefit from their use was demonstrated.[18] Thus they can be used to treat acute heart failure and continuing chest pain. If clinical features of heart failure persist or impaired left ventricular function is noted on echocardiography, an ACE inhibitor plus loop diuretic should be introduced, provided the patient is not hypotensive.

Calcium channel blockers are effective antianginal agents in diabetic subjects. They are metabolically neutral and do not worsen lipid profiles; they can be used to control angina post-AMI. There is no evidence of any beneficial or adverse effects of these agents on outcome post-AMI in diabetes, and they do not have a major role in acute management.

Progressive hypotension is an ominous sign, suggesting severe left ventricular dysfunction, causing reduced renal perfusion and progressive uraemia. Cardiogenic shock in a patient with diabetes should be treated as for normal subjects, but it is associated with a very poor prognosis.

How can the risk of future AMI be minimised?

The patient with diabetes, who emerges from coronary care, remains at high risk of future cardiac events. Mortality after one month and one year is double that for those without diabetes, and secondary prevention should form an essential part of long-term management.

Over the last 20 years, evidence from prospective trials has established beta-blockers, ACE inhibitors, and statins in secondary prevention in the general population. Unfortunately, many patients do not receive optimal therapy. A survey of 2583 patients attending Teaching or District General Hospitals in the United Kingdom showed inadequate documentation of known cardiovascular risk factors in many centres. One in five were not taking regular aspirin, only one in three were prescribed beta-blockers, and three-quarters had a total cholesterol of >5.2 mmol/litre.[19] In the following section the evidence supporting secondary prevention in diabetes is reviewed, and a protocol is suggested to provide optimal long-term management of patients post-AMI.

Advice on risk factor reduction

All patients with AMI, whether they have diabetes or not, should receive advice and support to stop smoking since this significantly reduces the risk of future ischaemic events. Lifestyle advice concerning exercise, diet and, where necessary, weight reduction should ideally be reinforced with a cardiac rehabilitation programme.

Beta-blockers

Beta-blockers have an established role in cardioprotection after AMI and may have particular advantages in diabetes. Several trials have studied the effect of beta-blockers on mortality post-AMI in patients with diabetes (Table 7.5). With the exception of one small study using pindolol, mortality was consistently reduced by beta-blockers.

Providing there are no contraindications, diabetic patients should be started on a cardioselective beta-blocker in the peri-infarct period. Concerns that they mask the symptoms of hypoglycaemia have been overstated since, in clinical practice, it is not a significant problem.

Lipid-lowering with statins

Evidence from several large trials with statins has clarified the role of lipid-lowering therapy in secondary prevention. The Scandinavian Simvastatin Survival Study (4S) trial provided clear evidence of benefit from lowering serum cholesterol.[25] Treatment was started if the serum cholesterol remained between 5.5 and 8.0 mmol/litre, despite dietary advice and the fasting serum triglycerides <2.5 mmol/litre. A recently published subgroup analysis of the 4S study has shown a 55% reduction in 202 patients with diabetes who were recruited into the trial (Table 7.6).[25] The Cholesterol and Recurrent Events (CARE) Trial enrolled 586 diabetic patients with a previous AMI out of a total cohort of 3573 patients.[26] Entry criteria were a myocardial infarction more than three but less than 20 months before randomisation, a total cholesterol <6.2 mmol/litre, and an LDL cholesterol of 3.0–4.5 mmol/litre. The major coronary event rate was 37% in those on placebo and 29% with pravastatin with similar benefit in the patients with diabetes (Table 7.6).

These studies suggest that the benefits of lipid-lowering therapy using statins are substantial, and that patients with diabetes benefit at least as much, if not more. As a routine, all patients with a suspected AMI should have their fasting cholesterol, LDL cholesterol, and triglycerides measured on admission. If this is not

Table 7.5 The effectiveness of beta-blockers in secondary prevention in patients with and without diabetes after AMI

Trial	Total no.	No. with diabetes	Duration (months)	Drug	Mortality Placebo (%)	Beta-blockers (%)
Norwegian Timolol Study[20]	1884	99	17	timolol	30.5	11.3
Kjekshus et al.[21]	1716	268	12	propranolol	23.4	10.2
BHAT Study[22]	3837	465	25	propranolol	14.4	9.3
Australian/Swedish Study[23]	529	36	48	pindolol	22.7	42.9
BIP Study Group[24]	14 417	2723	36	various	14.0	7.8

Table 7.6   Risk reduction in patients with diabetes given statins

Trial	Total nos.	Mean follow-up (months)	Patients with events		Risk reduction (%)
			placebo	HMG-CoA reductase inhibitor	
4S					
Non-diabetic	4242	64	578/2126	407/2116	32
Diabetic	202	64	44/97	24/105	55
CARE					
Non-diabetic	3573	60	437/1774	349/1799	23
Diabetic	586	60	81/304	25/282	25

possible, and AMI is confirmed, a fasting sample must be obtained between six weeks and three months after admission, because of the known effect of AMI in depressing serum cholesterol levels. Patients who have a fasting cholesterol of >5.5 mmol/litre or an LDL cholesterol >3.0 mmol/litre, despite dietary advice, should receive an HMG-CoA reductase inhibitor.

ACE inhibitors

ACE inhibitors have a proven role in the treatment of chronic heart failure in non-diabetic subjects, and benefits which have now been extended to patients with signs of heart failure or left ventricular dysfunction post-AMI where, for example, the International Study on Infarct Survival-4 (ISIS-4) trial reported a saving of five lives for every 1000 patients treated in the first month.[18]

The increased risk of heart failure post-AMI in patients with diabetes has been mentioned above. In the longer term, congestive cardiac failure is twice as common in middle-aged diabetic men and five times as common in women, and ACE inhibitors have an important role in management. Supporting data are limited but subset analysis of diabetic patients included in intervention trials (Survival after Ventricular Enlargement, SAVE trial)[27] and in chronic heart failure (Studies of Left Ventricular Dysfunction, SOLVD trials)[28] suggest similar benefit in reducing mortality and re-admission rates for heart failure compared with non-diabetics (Table 7.7). However, it should be noted that, even though ACE

Table 7.7 Subset analysis of patients with diabetes

Trial	n	Drug	Mean follow-up	Patients with events		Risk reduction (%)
				placebo	ACE	
SAVE						
Non diabetic	2231	C	37.4	448	335	24
Diabetic	492	C	37.4	137	109	17
SOLVD treatment trial						
Non-diabetic	1906	E	41	506	439	8
Diabetic	663	E	41	229	175	12
SOLVD prevention trial						
Non-diabetic	3581	E	37	399	345	3
Diabetic	647	E	37	119	88	10

Figures quoted the number of patients who experienced cardiovascular mortality, severe heart failure (needing hospitalisation), or a recurrent AMI. C = captopril; E = enalapril.

inhibitors probably improve prognosis, this remains significantly worse than for non-diabetics.

An algorithm for the acute management of AMI in patients with diabetes is shown in Figure 7.2.

Long-term follow-up

The patient with diabetes who successfully negotiates their time through the coronary care unit and medical ward is likely to be discharged on several different types of tablet, clutching a healthy eating diet plan and exercise programme, with a follow-up appointment for rehabilitation classes and appointments for medical and diabetic outpatients. A check up at four to six weeks is essential to review progress and check for symptoms of continuing angina or heart failure, and to assess medication for efficacy and side effects. Patients with postinfarction angina should be investigated with exercise testing according to local guidelines, with a view to offering angiography to those with limiting angina to assess their suitability for coronary revascularisation.

Revascularisation

Selected patients with diabetes benefit from revascularisation with either coronary artery bypass grafting (CABG) or coronary

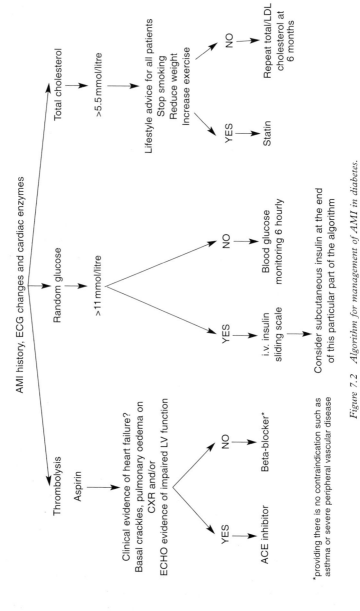

Figure 7.2 Algorithm for management of AMI in diabetes.

angioplasty (PTCA). The indications for revascularisation in diabetes are the same as for the general population, although a high index of suspicion is needed to pick up subtle clinical manifestations of ongoing cardiac ischaemia in patients with diabetes. Coronary vessels in diabetes tend to be more diffusely affected by atheroma than those of normal subjects, and this may partly explain the fact that the long-term prognosis after revascularisation is not generally as good as for non-diabetics. The Bypass Angioplasty Revascularisation (BARI) trial, the largest randomised comparison of bypass surgery and angioplasty in patients with multivessel disease, reported a five-year survival of 81% following CABG in patients with diabetes, significantly better than the 61% survival following angioplasty.[29] This relatively poor outcome of angioplasty was the result of a greater restenosis rate in diabetic subjects.

Based on the BARI trial, coronary artery bypass grafting is the preferred option in patients with diabetes with multivessel coronary disease. Provided patients are carefully selected, this operation is not associated with an increased perioperative mortality, although there may be a greater likelihood of postoperative wound infection. Metabolic control during cardiac surgery is discussed in Chapter 5.

Cerebrovascular disease

The prevalence of stroke is approximately doubled in people with diabetes, and some studies report an excess mortality compared with non-diabetics. Hypertension, which is common in type 2 diabetes, is a significant risk factor and, although long-term outcome studies are only recently being performed in diabetes, there is, however, strong evidence supporting antihypertensive therapy in stroke prevention in the general population. A recent study involving 583 elderly diabetic subjects showed that both fatal and non-fatal stroke and cardiac events were reduced by low-dose thiazide diuretic treatment of isolated systolic hypertension.

The Hypertension in Diabetes study has provided more evidence of the importance of blood pressure control in type 2 diabetes.[30] Patients with type 2 diabetes and hypertension (defined as BP $\geqslant 160/90$ in those previously untreated and $\geqslant 150/85$ in those on treatment) were randomised to "tight" blood pressure control (target $<150/85$ mmHg) with either a beta-blocker (atenolol) or an ACE inhibitor (captopril) as primary treatment, and a "less tight" control group (target <180/105 mmHg) in which beta-blockers or ACE inhibitors were avoided. Additional antihypertensive drugs, including frusemide, slow-release nifedipine, methyldopa, and prazosin, could be added if targets were not reached. Clinical end-points included fatal and non-fatal events, events related to diabetes, deaths related to diabetes and all cause mortality. Microvascular disease was assessed by serial retinal photography and urine albumin excretion. The key findings of the trial are shown in Table 7.8.

Table 7.8   Summary of the main findings of the Hypertension in Diabetes UKPDS trial[30]

Parameters	Tight BP control	Less tight BP control	% Risk reduction	P
Clinical				
Patients	758	390		
	(410 male)	(227 male)		
Mean entry BP	159/94	160/94		
Mean achieved BP	144/82	154/87		
Results				
All diabetes related end-points	259	170	24	0.0046
Diabetes related deaths	82	62	32	0.019
All cause mortality	134	83	18	0.17
Myocardial infarction	107	69	21	0.13
Stroke	38	34	44	0.013
Heart failure	21	24	56	0.0043
Microvascular complications	68	54	37	0.0092

There were no differences in outcome in the tight BP control group between those allocated to either a beta-blocker or ACE inhibitor. These results emphasise the importance of blood pressure control in type 2 diabetes in aiming for a target of 140/80 or less to reduce the risk of both macrovascular and microvascular complications. Another important clinical message is that combination therapy with three or more different antihypertensive drugs will be necessary in between one third and one half of patients. Other recently published trials, such as the Hypertension Optimal Treatment (HOT) trial,[31] have confirmed the benefit of intensive lowering of diastolic blood pressure to ≤80 mmHg, this was associated with a 51% reduction in major cardiovascular events compared with patients whose target diastolic blood pressure was ≤90 mmHg.

References

1 Diabetes and the heart. *Lancet* 1997;**350**(Suppl.1):1–32.

2 Yudkin JS, Oswald GA. Determinants of hospital admission and case fatality in diabetic patients with myocardial infarction. *Diabetes Care* 1988;**11**:351–8.

3 Tunbridge WMG. Factors contributing to the deaths of diabetics under fifty years of age. *Lancet* 1981;**i**:569–72.

4 UK Prospective Diabetes Survey VIII. Study design, progress and performance. *Diabetologia* 1991;**34**:877–90.

5 Orlander PR, Goff DC, Morrissey M *et al*. The relation of diabetes to the severity of acute myocardial infarction and post-myocardial infarction survival in Mexican-Americans and Non-Hispanic Whites. The Corpus Christi Heart Project. *Diabetes* 1994;**43**:897–902.

6 Fisher BM, Frier BM. Evidence for a specific heart muscle disease in humans. *Diabetic Med* 1990;**7**:478–89.

7 Herlitz J, Malmberg K, Karlson BW, Ryden L, Hjalmarson A. Mortality and morbidity during a five year follow-up of diabetics with myocardial infarction. *Acta Med Scand* 1988;**224**:31–8.

8 Vetter NJ, Strange RC, Adams W, Oliver MF. Initial metabolic and hormonal response to acute myocardial infarction. *Lancet* 1974;**i**: 284–8.

9 Gwilt DJ, Nattrass M, Pentecost BL. Use of low-dose insulin infusions in diabetics after myocardial infarction. *Br Med J* 1982;**285**:1402–4.

10 Malmberg K, Ryden L, Efendic S *et al*. Randomised trial of insulin-glucose infusion followed by subcutaneous insulin treatment in diabetic patients with acute myocardial infarction (DIGAMI study): Effects on mortality at 1 year. *J Am Coll Cardiol* 1995;**26**:57–65.

11 Malmberg K for the DIGAMI Study Group. Prospective randomised study of intensive insulin treatment on long term survival after acute myocardial infarction in patients with diabetes mellitus. *Br Med J* 1997;**314**:1512–15.

12 ISIS-2 Collaborative Group. Randomised trial of intravenous streptokinase, oral aspirin, both or neither among 17 187 cases of suspected acute myocardial infarction: ISIS-2. *Lancet* 1988;**ii**(8607): 349–60.

13 Lynch M, Gammage MD, Lamb P *et al*. Acute myocardial infarction in diabetic patients in the thrombolytic era. *Diabetic Med* 1994;**11**: 162–5.

14 Fibrinolytic Therapy Trialists' Collaborative Group. Indications for fibrinolytic therapy in suspected acute myocardial infarction: collaborative overview of early mortality and major morbidity results from all randomised trials of more than 1000 patients. *Lancet* 1994; **343**:311–22.

15 Hood S, Birnie D, Curzio JL *et al*. Wide variation in the use of thrombolysis among junior doctors in South and Central Scotland. *Health Bull* 1996;**54**:131–9.

16 Mahaffey KW, Granger CB, Toth CA *et al*. Diabetic retinopathy should not be a contraindication to thrombolytic therapy for acute

myocardial infarction: review of ocular haemorrhage incidence and location in the GUSTO-I trial. *J Am Coll Cardiol* 1997;**30**:1606–10.

17 Antiplatelet Trialists' Collaboration. Collaborative overview of randomised trials of antiplatelet therapy—I: Prevention of death, myocardial infarction and stroke by prolonged antiplatelet therapy in various categories of patient. *Br Med J* 1994;**308**:81–106.

18 ISIS-4 Collaborative Group. A randomised factorial trial assessing early oral captopril, oral mononitrate, and intravenous magnesium sulphate in 58 050 patients with suspected myocardial infarction: ISIS-4. *Lancet* 1995;**345**(8951):669–85.

19 Aspire Steering Group. A British Cardiac Society survey of the potential for the secondary prevention of coronary disease: ASPIRE (Action on Secondary Prevention through Intervention to Reduce Events). *Heart* 1996;**75**:334–42.

20 Norwegian Multicentre Study Group. Timolol-induced reduction in mortality and re-infarction in patients surviving acute myocardial infarction. *New Engl J Med* 1981;**304**:801–7.

21 Kjekshus J, Cilpin E, Cali G *et al.* Diabetic patients and beta-blockers after acute myocardial infarction. *Europ Heart J* 1990;**II**:43–50.

22 Beta-blocker Heart Attack Trial Research Group. A randomised trial of propanolol in patients with acute myocardial infarction. *J Am Med Ass* 1982;**247**:1707–14.

23 Australian and Swedish Pindolol Study Group. The effect of pindolol on the two year mortality after complicated myocardial infarction. *Europ Heart J* 1983;**4**:367–75.

24 Bezafibrate Infarction Prevention (BIP) Study Group. Usefulness of beta-blocker therapy in patients with non-insulin-dependent diabetes mellitus and coronary artery disease. *Am J Cardiol* 1996;**77**:1273–7.

25 Scandinavian Simvastatin Survival Study (4S). Cholesterol lowering improves prognosis of diabetic patients with coronary heart disease. *Diabetes Care* 1997;**20**:614–20.

26 Sacks FM, Pfeffer MA, Moye LA *et al.* The effect of pravastatin on coronary events after myocardial infarction in patients with average cholesterol levels. *New Engl J Med* 1996;**335**:1001–9.

27 SAVE. Uniformity of benefit in the SAVE study: subgroup analysis. *Europ Heart J* 1994;**15**:2–8.

28 SOLVD. Diabetes mellitus, a predictor of morbidity and mortality in the studies of left ventricular dysfunction trials and registry. *Am J Cardiol* 1996;**77**:1017–20.

29 Bypass Angioplasty Revascularisation Investigation (BARI) Investigators. Comparison of coronary bypass surgery with angioplasty in patients with multivessel disease. *New Engl J Med* 1996;**335**:217–25.

30 UKPDS 38. Tight blood pressure control and the risk of macrovascular and microvascular complications in type 2 diabetes. *Br Med J* 1998;**317**:703–13.

31 Hansson L, Zanchetti A, Carruthers SG *et al.* Effect of intensive blood pressure lowering and low-dose aspirin in patients with hypertension: principal results of the Hypertension Optimal Treatment (HOT) randomised trial. *Lancet* 1998;**351**:1755–62.

8 The diabetic foot

Foot ulcers are a common and serious complication of diabetes. Community surveys in the UK suggest an overall prevalence of 3–5% with most minor lesions cared for by patients themselves or the Primary Care team. They usually present as emergencies as a result of superimposed soft tissue or bone infection, or because of peripheral gangrene or rest pain. Early assessment and appropriate treatment plays a major part in limiting tissue damage and reducing the risk of amputation. Most patients with acute diabetic foot ulcers are admitted directly onto surgical or health care of the elderly wards, even in hospitals that provide a specialist foot clinic service, and these account for 20% of all diabetes-related admissions. Average length of stay varies between two and four weeks, depending on the site and nature of the ulcer, and treatment is therefore expensive. The risk of amputation is 15-fold higher than in non-diabetics, with half of all non-traumatic lower limb amputations performed in diabetics. Overall risk of foot ulceration and amputation increases with age and is more common with lower social class and in male sex. This chapter describes the aetiology, assessment, and management of diabetic foot ulcers.

What causes foot ulcers?

Ulcers result from injury or trauma to a foot that is "at-risk" because of sensory loss from diabetic peripheral neuropathy (neuropathic), impaired blood supply from peripheral vascular disease or microvascular disease (ischaemic), or a combination of these (neuro-ischaemic). Most patients have a combination of neuropathy and vascular disease, but it is useful to discuss the principles of management of purely "neuropathic" or "ischaemic" ulcers.

Neuropathic ulcers

The overall prevalence of clinically detectable peripheral neuropathy was found to be 28% in unselected patients attending

149

hospital diabetes clinics in the United Kingdom.[1] The risk of neuropathy increases with duration of diabetes and, of those with diabetes for 25 years, 50% suffer from it.[2] Poor glycaemic control, male sex, smoking, and tallness are also recognised risk factors for neuropathy. In contrast to patients with type 1 diabetes, who do not have neuropathy at onset of their diabetes, 10% of those with type 2 diabetes do, and occasionally a foot ulcer may be the first presentation of diabetes as shown in the following case history.

Case Study 19

A 54-year-old man was referred as a surgical emergency with a foot ulcer which had become secondarily infected. On examination he had a deep ulcer over his first metatarsal head, with swelling and redness of the forefoot and localised crepitus. The ulcer was painless and the admitting physician found reduced sensation in both feet to the mid-calves, to both pinprick and vibration sense. Urinalysis confirmed glycosuria, and random blood glucose was 17.4 mmol/litre. On reassessing the history the patient admitted to having had thirst and occasional nocturia for at least six months. Full assessment revealed reduced visual acuity in the left eye, with bilateral background retinopathy and early maculopathy in the left eye. He also had + + protein in routine urinalysis and a raised serum creatinine of 130 μmol/litre.

Two important clinical messages arise from the above case; first, patients may present with a foot ulcer as the first clinically recognised feature of diabetes and, secondly, such patients often have other complications and require careful assessment, including fundoscopy through dilated pupils (see Chapter 9).

Peripheral neuropathy, which is found in over 80% of patients with diabetic foot ulceration, is an important aetiological factor for a number of reasons (Table 8.1).

Neuropathic ulceration occurs most commonly on weight-bearing areas of the foot, especially over the metatarsal heads, first hallux, and heels. Deformities such as claw toes, hallux valgus or rigidus, or previous amputation increase pressure over specific areas of the feet. If the patient continues to walk, callus accumulates over pressure points and a vicious cycle of increasing pressure and further callus formation traumatises underlying tissues until ulceration occurs. In effect, walking on hard callus is like having a stone in your shoe. Small capillary haemorrhages can sometimes

Table 8.1   Consequences of peripheral sensory neuropathy in diabetes

Change	Consequence
Insensitivity	Increased risk of trauma
	Patients may wear inappropriate poorly fitting shoes
Small muscle wasting	Clawing of the toes with displacement of metatarsal fat pads leading to excessive pressure over the heads of the metatarsal bones
	Abnormal pressure over the metatarsal heads with callus over pressure points
Autonomic neuropathy	Loss of sympathetic innervation to sweat glands
	Dry cracked skin

be seen within callus, and are an important physical sign because they are associated with a high probability of ulceration.

Often ulcers can appear small and insignificant in a central area of callus, but once this has been debrided, there is often a much larger area of tissue damage underneath. Patients need to be warned about this possibility so that the chiropodist is not unfairly blamed for "causing the ulcer".

Another common site for neuropathic ulceration is over the upper aspect of the proximal interphalangeal joint, particularly associated with clawing of toes. Patients often have difficulty finding shoes which are sufficiently deep to accommodate the deformity and pressure from footwear causes the ulceration.

The neuropathic heel is also vulnerable to pressure, particularly in the bed-bound. Prevention is always better than cure, and any patient with diabetes, who needs hospital treatment which involves bed rest or immobility, should be assessed for signs of neuropathy (Box 8.1).

Box 8.1   Clinical features of the "at risk neuropathic foot"

- Reduced or absent pinprick perception (to Neurotips or equivalent)
- Reduced or absent perception of cottonwool
- Reduced or absent vibration perception
- Absent ankle jerks

During the admission patients with "at-risk feet" should have their feet examined daily for blisters or skin breakdown, over the heels in particular. Measures should be used to minimise pressure, such as heel protection with padded dressings or the use of foam leg-troughs to elevate the heel.[3]

It is important to emphasise that neuropathy alone does not lead to the development of foot ulcers without some form of trauma, either related to pressure, ill-fitting shoes or, occasionally, to more dramatic causes as is illustrated in case study 20. This case illustrates how rapidly infection can complicate skin injury in the diabetic foot (see below), and how neuropathy can delay presentation because the patient feels little, if any, discomfort and assumes nothing is wrong. Identification of patients with "at-risk" feet as a result of neuropathy is an important part of routine diabetic care. Once identified, such patients need education about foot care, including the need to have their feet measured before buying new shoes, together with regular chiropody.

Case Study 20

A 53-year-old woman with a five-year history of type 2 diabetes was walking in her sitting room with no shoes. She trod on a drawing pin and, because of peripheral neuropathy, only noticed this had happened when she saw blood on the carpet. She removed the pin, and, since there were no signs other than the small puncture mark and no pain, she thought no more of the episode. Two days later she felt a slight throbbing sensation between her toes and noticed that her foot was swollen and red. She saw her GP later the same day who arranged urgent admission. On arrival she had marked erythema and swelling of her forefoot with a fluctuant area in the first webspace. All peripheral pulses were palpable, although marked sensory neuropathy was noted and the foot was only minimally painful. She was started on intravenous broad spectrum antibiotics and required urgent surgical drainage of an abscess in her first and second web space. The admission lasted three weeks, and it took six weeks for the wound to finally heal.

Vascular disease

People with diabetes often have peripheral vascular disease. Intermittent claudication is four and six times more common in diabetic men and women respectively, and at diagnosis up to 20% of people with type 2 diabetes have absent or reduced foot pulses. Vascular disease complicates up to 75% of diabetic foot ulcers, usually with peripheral neuropathy (neuroischaemic ulcers), whilst pure ischaemic ulcers account for about 10%.

It is well recognised that vascular disease is more severe and extensive in diabetes and typically affects the three major vessels below the knee. A common finding is reasonably good iliofemoral vessels that "peter out" below the knee causing critical ischaemia of the foot. Peripheral vascular disease plays an important role in the pathogenesis of foot ulcers and is a strong predictor of the need for amputation.[4]

Referral to hospital is usually precipitated by worsening symptoms of claudication affecting the calves, thighs, or buttocks, or by rest pain that is often worse at night as is shown in the case history below.

Case Study 21

A 74-year-old man with diet-controlled type 2 diabetes was referred urgently because of increasing pain in his left forefoot and discolouration of his big toe. He had a cold foot with pregangrenous changes in the hallux and very poor capillary return in the other toes. No pulses were palpable below the femoral, and it was not possible to detect an arterial Doppler signal from either of his foot pulses. He was admitted for pain control and an urgent arteriogram which showed an occluded popliteal artery aneurysm and single-vessel run-off via the common peroneal artery below the knee. The following day he underwent local vein grafting with restoration of arterial flow to the foot.

Critical ischaemia is signalled by the development of rest pain and is an indication for urgent assessment. There is often, but not always, a history of previous intermittent claudication, and there may be one or several indolent foot ulcers usually around the periphery of the foot.

The appearance of an ischaemic foot is very different to a neuropathic one. The foot is cold, the skin atrophic, and there may be loss of hair over the lower half of the leg. Nails may show atrophic changes. Callus may be absent over pressure points, even in the presence of neuropathy, because of poor skin oxygenation. Capillary perfusion is usually sluggish and the foot may be pale or cyanosed. Venous return is slow, with "guttering" of veins on the dorsum of the foot, and the foot becomes "marbled" in appearance on elevation of the leg. The foot then becomes hyperaemic when lowered, owing to the effects of tissue hypoxia (Buerger's sign).

In contrast to the neuropathic foot, pulses are usually weak or impalpable but, because of the distribution of atherosclerosis in diabetes, popliteal pulses may be easily felt. Full non-invasive assessment of the arteries of the foot with Doppler ultrasound should be performed. The failure to identify any signal (as in the above case) indicates critical limb-threatening ischaemia and the need for urgent radiological assessment. If a Doppler signal is identified, it is useful to estimate the ankle-brachial pressure index. A sphygmomanometer cuff is placed above the ankle and inflated until the Doppler signal disappears. The cuff should then be gradually deflated until the signal just returns giving a measure of ankle systolic pressure. Comparison with the brachial systolic pressure gives a ratio which should be >1.0. Values <0.6 indicate severe ischaemia. It is common not to be able to occlude the Doppler signal in the foot, despite high cuff pressures, because of the medial calcification present in the arterial wall of many diabetic patients. Under these circumstances the ankle-brachial pressure index can be misleading and should be interpreted in the context of other clinical features.

Ischaemic foot ulceration usually occurs in patients with other vascular disease and it is very important to examine the entire cardiovascular system for signs of poor left ventricular function, cardiac failure, or atrial fibrillation.

When does the diabetic foot need hospital admission?

It is useful to have a simple classification of diabetic foot ulcers which can be used to judge the level of clinical intervention that is likely to be needed (Table 8.2).[5] Hospital admission is necessary for infected ⩾grade 2 ulcers to determine the extent of the ulcer, relieve pressure with bed rest, control infection and, where necessary, assess the vascular supply. Admission also enables diabetic control to be assessed and optimised and other risk factors for macrovascular disease to be treated.

The site and size of the ulcer should be documented and the peripheral pulses carefully palpated. Signs of deep infection, including tracks from the ulcer base, areas of fluctuance or purulent discharge should be sought, together with a general assessment of the patient's condition. Deep foot infection may precipitate

154

Table 8.2   Classification and management of diabetic foot ulcers

Grade	Description	Management
Outpatient		
Grade 0	At-risk foot	Education, chiropody, footwear
Grade 1	Superficial ulcer	Pressure relief, chiropody, dressings
Grade 2	Deep ulcer, no osteomyelitis	Pressure relief, chiropody, dressings
Inpatient		
Grade 2	Deep ulcer + infection No osteomyelitis	Pressure relief, chiropody, dressings, antibiotics
Grade 3	Deep ulcer Osteomyelitis or abscess	Pressure relief, chiropody, dressings, antibiotics. Often need surgical debridement
Grade 4	Localised gangrene	Pressure relief, antibiotics, consider arteriogram May require revascularisation ± local amputation
Grade 5	Extensive gangrene	Below or above knee amputation

ketoacidosis in patients with type 1 diabetes. Initial investigations should include microbiological swabs, blood cultures, and foot X-rays for possible osteomyelitis.

Oedema should be treated with bed rest and elevation of the affected limb. Prophylactic heparinisation (5000 units b.d.) should be considered. Good diabetic control is probably important for optimisation of neutrophil function and host defences against infection. It may be necessary to transfer a patient with type 2 diabetes onto insulin to achieve this.

Broad spectrum intravenous antibiotics (see below) should be started if there are signs of infection, and an early surgical opinion should be sought if there is abscess formation, since drainage is limb-saving in some cases. Management of diabetes during such surgery is discussed in Chapter 5.

Intravenous antibiotics should be continued until there has been a clinical response, and it may be necessary to modify the regimen in the light of cultures. With clinical improvement, patients can be transferred to oral antibiotics, which should be continued for a week after signs of infection have resolved. With associated osteomyelitis, oral antibiotics should be continued for at least six weeks, with progress assessed on clinical and radiological grounds. Progression of bone disease is an indication for surgical review and debridement of infected bone.

Optimal management of most foot ulcers involves joint management between diabetes and surgical teams and, once improvement has occurred, continued nursing care with the support of the chiropodist and podiatrist as appropriate is essential. Throughout such a hospital admission it is vital to remember the other foot is also likely to be "at-risk". Regular examination and advice on foot care and heel protection are essential to prevent ulceration of the other foot.

Some of these general issues will be discussed in more detail below.

Management of the non-infected neuropathic ulcer

Treatment is based on reducing pressure by frequent (weekly or biweekly) chiropody to remove callus from the edges of the ulcer. Patients can usually be kept ambulant by the use of lightweight plaster casts or removable Scotchcast boots,[6] which allow a "cut-out" window to be incorporated at the site of the ulcer. With such treatment, provided secondary infection does not develop, most neuropathic ulcers heal over a period of several weeks. Once healed, patients need intensive education about foot care. Appropriate footwear with pressure-redistributing insoles should be provided in certain cases to reduce the risk of future ulceration. Continuing chiropody is mandatory.

Infection in diabetic foot ulcers

Infection is the commonest reason for emergency admission of diabetic foot ulcers as the following case illustrates.

Case Study 22

A 56-year-old man with type 2 diabetes had been attending a hospital clinic with a foot ulcer for two months. He had reduced sensation to pinprick, light touch, and vibration on both feet, but had easily palpable foot pulses. He had developed an ulcer under his 2nd and 3rd metatarsal heads, which had been treated with a pressure relieving Scotchcast boot, regular dressings, and chiropody. The ulcer was slowly responding to treatment. Five days before attending clinic he had felt generally unwell, with anorexia, malaise, and episodic sweats, and had noted that his foot had become rather more swollen than usual. His diabetes, which was normally well controlled on diet and tablets, had deteriorated with persistent glycosuria. He saw his general practitioner who started him on oral flucloxacillin. At the diabetic foot clinic five days later he was unwell with a fever, and marked swelling and redness of the foot. The ulcer base showed a sinus track extending into the tissues of the mid-foot. He was admitted directly for bed rest, intravenous broad spectrum antibiotics, and he required urgent surgical drainage of pus with laying open of the sinus track. During the acute admission, insulin treatment was temporarily used to control hyperglycaemia. The admission lasted 27 days. The wound took a further three months to heal.

About 60% of infections start in the web spaces, 30% around the nails, and 10% occur as a result of puncture wounds, either traumatic or from neuropathic ulceration. Infection usually presents as a hot, swollen, red foot, although these signs may be minimal in some patients. With neuropathy, pain and tenderness may be absent. The lack of pain may falsely reassure the patient (and sometimes the doctor), and this can delay appropriate referral. Pressure from continued walking may also cause more rapid spread of infection within the foot and lead to extensive soft tissue damage.

Infections are usually polymicrobial with an average isolate of between two and four organisms per ulcer,[7] although it is often not clear which are pathogenic and which commensals. Superficial infection is often due to *Staphylococcus aureus* or *Streptococcus pyogenes*, whereas gram-negative bacteria, such as *Escherichia coli*, *Proteus* or *Klebsiella* spp., and anaerobic organisms, such as *Bacteroides*, *Peptostreptococcus* and *Clostridium* spp., are often found in deep foot infection with osteomyelitis.

Treatment with antibiotics

Antibiotic treatment must be *broad spectrum*, covering both aerobic and anaerobic organisms, to cope with the range of potential infecting organisms; the choice of flucloxacillin in the above case was insufficient. Useful antibiotic regimens are shown in Box 8.2.

Superficial infections can be treated with oral antibiotics with frequent review in outpatients, but deeper infections usually require admission with intravenous antibiotics until the infection responds. Oral antibiotics can then be continued until signs of infection have settled.

Deeper infection should be suspected if there is a purulent discharge, crepitus, or sinuses extending into the foot. Deep foot

---

Box 8.2 Appropriate antibiotic regimens for infected diabetic foot ulcers

Monotherapy
- Clindamycin: Good bone penetration; useful in osteomyelitis
- Augmentin: Spectrum includes aerobic and anaerobic organisms

Combination therapy
- Clindamycin and ciprofloxacin: Good bone and tissue penetration; useful in osteomyelitis
- I.v. ampicillin/flucloxacillin and oral metronidazole: Standard regimen for hospitalised patients
- Erythromycin/metronidazole: Alternative in patients with penicillin allergy
- Cefuroxime/metronidazole: Alternative in patients with penicillin allergy

---

infections are often complicated by osteomyelitis. This usually affects the phalanges or the metatarsal bones, and produces a characteristic tense brawny oedema around the affected site, often associated with sinus tracks. Bone destruction, especially if involving the phalanges leads to typical "instability" of the digit. Osteomyelitis should be assumed if bone is exposed or it is possible to "probe to bone". Such deep probing should also be used to obtain material for microbiological culture. Foot X-rays should be taken where osteomyelitis is suspected. Radiographic bone destruction may not become apparent for several weeks, and X-rays should be repeated every two to four weeks, particularly if sinuses or localised oedema persist despite antibiotics. MRI scanning is more sensitive in demonstrating early bone involvement. Other scans may help: ^{99m}Tc bone scanning is sensitive for osteomyelitis, but increased uptake is also seen in an early Charcot foot (see below) and may cause diagnostic difficulties. Indium-labelled white cell scanning is also sensitive in picking up early infection but has limitations in differentiating bone from soft tissue involvement.

Osteomyelitis affecting a digit or metatarsal head often responds to a prolonged course of oral antibiotics often extending over 6–12 weeks. A combination of clindamycin and ciprofloxacin (or equivalent) is particularly effective and may lead to healing in 80%

of cases.[8] Surgical debridement remains an option in managing osteomyelitis and should be considered where bone destruction progresses despite conservative measures.

Surgical intervention

The extent and severity of infection and the adequacy of vascular supply determine the role of surgery in the management of diabetic foot ulcers. As discussed above, superficial infection usually responds to broad spectrum antibiotics alone but, if infection has spread into deep compartments in the foot, surgical drainage and debridement is usually required to remove collections and associated devitalised tissue, including bone. This must be performed as an emergency to limit progressive tissue damage, even if there is concern about the arterial supply to the limb. In this event urgent assessment of the circulation should be organised in the postoperative period with a view to revascularisation.

All patients with a foot ulcer need thorough assessment of their peripheral arterial circulation. Clinical and Doppler assessment have been described above. Where there are features of severe ischaemia, further assessment is necessary. If available, colour Duplex scanning is a useful non-invasive method of assessing stenotic lesions above the knee, but is operator-dependent and less effective for identifying severity of disease below the knee. In most centres arteriography is the investigation of choice in a severely ischaemic limb. This should be arranged in consultation with the vascular surgical team, particularly if angioplasty is considered because of the small risk of arterial dissection or rupture during the procedure. The indications for arteriography are shown in Box 8.3.

To minimise the risk of contrast-induced nephrotoxicity with angiography, care should be taken to maintain hydration during and after the procedure (see Chapter 6).

Peripheral transluminal angioplasty is a useful technique in the management of peripheral vascular disease. It is performed under local anaesthetic and involves the introduction of a catheter into the target femoral artery with the use of a Seldinger technique. A guidewire is passed across the stenosis or occluded segment. Once this is in place, an angioplasty balloon is positioned across the stenosis and inflated to 6–12 atmospheres. Once complete, a repeat angiogram is performed to check the vessel has a satisfactory lumen.

Box 8.3 Indications for arteriography

- Claudication affecting lifestyle
- Severe claudication
- Rest pain
- Gangrene
- Ischaemic, non-healing ulcers
- Preoperatively
- Graft stenosis or compromise

The technique is suitable for stenotic (>70%) or short (<3 cm) occlusive lesions in the iliac, femoral, or popliteal vessels, and can be highly effective in salvaging a critically ischaemic foot as is demonstrated in the case history.

Case Study 23

A 75-year-old man with a four-year history of type 2 diabetes was referred urgently because of dusky discolouration of his right second and third toes, with associated pain in his forefoot, which had been getting worse over three weeks. On examination, he had cold feet with obvious trophic nail changes, and there were ischaemic changes in the affected toes which were pregangrenous. His foot pulses were impalpable, the popliteal pulse was weak, and there was a loud bruit over the femoral artery of the affected side. Doppler studies were obtained showing an ankle-brachial index of 0.6, consistent with severe ischaemia. Urgent arteriography showed a 3 cm stenosis in the lower superficial femoral artery with single vessel run-off in the calf. A subsequent angioplasty was attempted with successful recanalisation and improvement in symptoms of rest pain, but the toes did not improve and became gangrenous. Since the toes were clearly demarcated, it was decided to allow them to autoamputate. He was discharged with appropriate footwear and instructions for follow-up in the diabetic foot clinic.

Complications of angioplasty are uncommon but include re-stenosis, distal embolisation of atheromatous material, and dissection. The latter can lead to acute arterial occlusion and may require emergency surgical bypass grafting.

The decision to perform vascular surgery depends on the anatomy of occlusive disease, the risk of surgery, and the potential for rehabilitation. Where there is severe disease of major proximal vessels, or a long occlusion of the superficial femoral artery, aortofemoral or femoropopliteal grafting can be very effective, with similar patency rates to those in non-diabetics.[9] Unfortunately the predilection of atheroma to affect the vessels below the knee means that proximal surgery may be less effective in treating foot ulcers, because of poor run-off into the calf vessels. Vascular surgical techniques now allow distal grafting, usually from the popliteal artery to a suitable patent artery at the ankle. Autologous vein grafts are the most satisfactory material with prosthetic materials being a poor alternative. Such surgery can salvage limbs that would otherwise require amputation. Although technically demanding, distal grafting can achieve three-year limb salvage rates of 65%.[10]

It is important to remember that patients with diabetes and peripheral vascular disease who require bypass surgery are likely to have extensive vascular disease elsewhere. This is reflected in figures showing that the perioperative myocardial infarction rate was 7.3% in 191 patients at a regional surgical unit in Scotland.[11] Angina was a strong predictor of risk. Careful preoperative assessment is required in all patients who need vascular surgery, particularly to optimise their cardiorespiratory status (Chapter 5).

Gangrene in the neuropathic foot

Gangrene can complicate the neuropathic foot, usually as a result of secondary infection as is illustrated in the following case history.

Case Study 24

A 28-year-old man with long-standing type 1 diabetes was moving some house bricks in his garden. Peripheral neuropathy had been noted at several annual reviews and he had received appropriate advice about footcare but, on this occasion, was only wearing slippers. He dropped the brick which landed on the base of his right fifth toe causing a small laceration and some local bruising. Because the injury was virtually painless, he did not think it was too serious and only became concerned two days later, when he noted local redness and swelling, extending from the base of the toe onto the plantar aspect of the foot. He saw his GP who prescribed flucloxacillin and told him to rest. Two days later he was no better and was concerned that the fifth toe had become discoloured. He was referred as an emergency to hospital where he was noted to have a gangrenous fifth toe, cellulitis, and extensive tissue necrosis extending into the mid-foot. He was started on intravenous ampicillin, flucloxacillin, and metronidazole, and required urgent surgical debridement with amputation of the fifth toe on the day of admission.

The wound gradually healed over four months, when he remained ambulant by using a Scotchcast boot. He was supplied with bespoke shoes following healing.

In this case, secondary infection caused occlusion of the paired digital arteries to the fifth toe with resulting gangrene. This situation may occur despite easily palpable major foot pulses. With extensive deep infection, it is necessary to surgically debride necrotic tissue and drain pockets of pus and, unlike the situation with the ischaemic foot (see below), the affected toe(s) are best amputated, since the good blood supply should ensure rapid healing of the wound. Appropriate antibiotics should be continued during the post-operative period until signs of infection have resolved.

Microembolic disease

Occasionally atheromatous material may dislodge from proximal vessels and embolise to small vessels in the periphery. The following case history is typical.

Case Study 25

A 64-year-old man with a seven-year history of type 2 diabetes presented with acute onset of severe pain in several toes on both feet. He had been a long-term smoker but had no previous symptoms of claudication or rest pain. His diabetes was controlled with diet alone. On examination he had multiple small ischaemic ulcers on his toes. He had an absent posterior tibial arterial pulse in both legs, but both dorsalis pedis pulses were present. There was a right femoral bruit. Cardiovascular examination was otherwise normal. He was in sinus rhythm.

A diagnosis of microvascular embolic disease was made and he was admitted for further assessment. He was started on aspirin, 300 mg daily, and received a course of Iloprost by daily intravenous infusion. His analgesic requirements fell markedly towards the end of the treatment period and he was discharged home with follow-up in the diabetes foot clinic. There was gradual healing of all ischaemic ulcers, with the exception of established dry gangrene of the left fifth toe which eventually autoamputated.

Iloprost is a prostacyclin analogue (prostaglandin I_2 analogue) which dilates peripheral arterioles and venules, reduces platelet aggregation, and activates fibrinolysis. It is usually administered by daily intravenous infusion for between 14 and 28 days. Randomised controlled trials have shown a reduction in major amputation over six months, suggesting that it might have a role in patients with severe peripheral vascular disease who are unsuitable for angioplasty or bypass surgery.[12]

Control of diabetes

As with all intercurrent illness, foot infections usually cause insulin resistance and hyperglycaemia, which might impair neutrophil function and lower natural immunity. Control of hyperglycaemia is an essential part of management: in patients already on insulin, an increased dose (sometimes a doubling or more of the total daily dose) is usually necessary. This is best achieved using the patient's normal regimen (e.g. twice daily or basal bolus regimen), which should be reviewed and adjusted at the end of each day, according to capillary blood glucose measurements (see Chapter 2). Increases of 10–20% of the total daily dose are usually needed if blood glucose exceeds the target range of 7–11 mmol/litre. Patients on once daily insulin usually need more frequent injections and a short-term basal bolus regimen should be used.

In those on diet or tablets, regular monitoring of capillary blood glucose is important during the acute admission. It is usually best to use insulin if the blood glucose is consistently >11 mmol/litre and a basal bolus regimen (Chapter 2) offers most flexibility. An initial daily dose of 0.3–0.5 units/kg should be estimated and divided into four injections as shown in Box 8.4. If the patient is vomiting, or it proves difficult to control the blood glucose with subcutaneous insulin, an intravenous glucose/insulin/potassium regimen (Chapter 2) should be used.

Management on discharge

Patients with neuropathic foot ulcers should only be discharged once signs of infection have resolved, the ulcer base is clean and granulating, and arrangements for dressings in the community have been made. It is also important to provide appropriate footwear. Patients with plantar ulcers usually need a lightweight plaster or Scotchcast boot, whilst those with ulcers or amputation sites in

Box 8.4 Insulin regimen for inpatients with diabetic foot

Regimen for 70 kg man normally on gliclazide 80 mg b.d., admitted with an infected neuropathic foot ulcer, with fasting capillary blood sugars 13–15 mmol/litre and post-prandial capillary blood sugars 18–25 mmol/ litre.

- Initial daily insulin dose: 0.5 × 70, approximately 35 units
- Suggested basal bolus regimen: 60% soluble insulin (3 equal doses), 40% isophane

	Pre-breakfast (units)	Pre-lunch (units)	Pre-evening meal (units)	Pre-bed (units)
Soluble insulin	8	8	8	—
Isophane	—	—	—	12

- Doses should be adjusted daily depending on pre-meal capillary blood glucose measurements.

non-weight bearing areas should have temporary (Neoprene) shoes to accommodate dressings. Frequent review is needed, ideally by a specialist foot clinic supported by chiropody and orthotist services.

Large surgical wounds resulting from debridement of infection in a neuropathic foot, particularly those on the dorsal aspect of the foot, might be suitable for split-skin grafting to hasten wound healing. A recent alternative is Dermagraft, a preparation of cultured neonatal foreskin fibroblasts grown on a supporting mesh, which is applied to a clean granulating wound weekly for eight weeks. Initial reports have shown improved healing rates.[13]

Charcot foot

A Charcot foot is an uncommon complication of severe peripheral neuropathy that can cause gross bony deformity with a high risk of ulceration. The pathogenesis is poorly understood but a combination of factors are probably involved. Neuropathy is associated with increased blood flow to the foot, which can predispose to thinning of the bones of the tarsus, termed diabetic osteopaenia. Minor trauma can cause a stress fracture in a tarsal bone which, because the foot is painless, goes unnoticed by the patient. Continued walking causes more bone destruction, fragmentation and, ultimately, bone remodelling, leading to deformity of the bones of the foot. Early signs can be misinterpreted as local infection as is shown in the following case history.

Case Study 26

A 45-year-old man with long-standing diabetes presented to his GP with a two-week history of aching discomfort in his left foot. He had also noted swelling and redness over the arch of the foot, which meant that his usual shoes no longer fitted; he had therefore been wearing training shoes. His GP requested urgent hospital referral for suspected cellulitis. On assessment in the admissions ward, the foot was hot and swollen with some erythema over the dorsal aspect, although no portal of entry for local infection was identified. A marked peripheral neuropathy was confirmed with loss of pinprick and vibration sensation in both feet extending to the mid-calf. Subsequent biosthesiometer readings exceeded 50 V in both feet. He was afebrile with a normal white count, ESR (erythrocyte sedimentation rate), and CRP (C-reactive protein). Plain X-rays were normal but a ^{99m}Tc bone scan showed marked increased uptake in the mid-foot; Charcot arthropathy was diagnosed.

Occasionally, it can be difficult to distinguish acute bone infection from an early Charcot foot. Inflammatory markers, such as ESR or CRP, can help since these are usually raised in extensive osteomyelitis, and normal in Charcot foot. Where there is doubt, indium-labelled white-cell scanning is useful; a Charcot arthropathy gives a negative scan.

Treatment of an evolving Charcot arthropathy is difficult. Some doctors recommend rest with a period of non-weight bearing, and others suggest immobilisation in a plaster cast for 6–12 weeks, followed by gradual mobilisation after provision of appropriate footwear with moulded insoles. Bisphosphonates have reduced pain and swelling in uncontrolled trials[14] and controlled trials are currently in progress.

Severe peripheral neuropathy also predisposes to bony injury which can lead to patients seeking advice from emergency departments as is seen in the following case.

Case Study 27

A 63-year-old amateur ornithologist had diabetes diagnosed in 1981. He had started insulin in 1991 because of worsening control on diet and tablets. He had laser photocoagulation for severe diabetic retinopathy but had no symptoms relating to his feet.

Whilst on a bird watching holiday, he stepped heavily from a quay onto a boat and noted sudden discomfort in his right foot. Later that day he had some difficulty removing his shoe because the foot had swollen. He attended the local casualty department who X-rayed the foot and found fractures of his 2nd, 3rd, and 4th metatarsal heads. He was advised to rest and provided with elbow crutches. At his diabetic clinic appointment, repeat X-rays confirmed partially healed fractures. A severe peripheral neuropathy was noted with biosthesiometer voltage over 50 V in both feet. He was referred to the orthotist for shoe fitting.

One year later, he presented urgently to the diabetes foot clinic with a two-week history of pain in his left foot. He was sure that he had not injured the foot, but did admit to getting caught in a "bog" whilst bird watching and having to struggle to extricate his foot. The pain developed 24 hours after this episode. Plain X-rays showed fractures of the 2nd and 3rd metatarsal bones. He was advised to give up bird watching! The fractures eventually healed after he was put in a walking plantar boot. He has subsequently developed Charcot deformity in that foot.

Fracture of metatarsal bones is usually treated conservatively with rest and immobilisation in the expectation that they will heal. Such patients are at considerable risk of neuropathic ulceration and require education about foot care.

Amputation

Lower limb amputation is 15 times more common in patients with diabetes than in the general population.[15] Amputation should be reserved for patients with severe ischaemia associated with inoperable vascular disease and rest pain. In such clinical situations attempts at more limited resections are almost always unsuccessful. Removing the leg in pieces is never a satisfactory management plan. Occasionally severe infection with extensive tissue necrosis of the mid-foot or heel, or severe unresponsive osteomyelitis, requires primary amputation. The perioperative cardiovascular risks are similar to those for vascular bypass surgery and the operation should be undertaken with an experienced anaesthetist in a patient whose cardiovascular status has been optimised preoperatively.

The long-term outlook following amputation for severe vascular disease is not encouraging. Median life expectancy has been reported as 22 months,[16] and there is a 50% chance that a diabetic amputee will either lose the other limb or die within three years of the primary amputation.

Other problems associated with neuropathy

Although foot ulcers are the most common problem associated with neuropathy, several clinical syndromes are recognised as acute manifestations of neuropathy. These may present to general medical, neurological, or orthopaedic departments, and are described below.

Painful peripheral neuropathy

Distal sensorimotor neuropathy may be associated with pain in a stocking distribution. It is variously described as burning, like pins and needles, or increased sensitivity to normal stimuli, (allodynia). These symptoms tend to be continuous and are typically worse at night: sleep is often disturbed. Weight loss is often a prominent feature. The natural history of peripheral neuropathic pain is for it to gradually resolve over 12 to 18 months; it is replaced by sensory loss with an increased risk of neuropathic foot ulceration, although clinical experience suggests some patients run a much more protracted course. Optimal diabetic control is the only intervention shown to slow the rate of progression of neuropathy. Symptomatic control can be achieved in most cases using tricyclic antidepressants such as amitryptilene or imipramine at night.[17] Other more "modern" antidepressants, such as the serotonin reuptake inhibitors (SSRIs), do not work. Where tricyclic agents do not work or are too sedating, anticonvulsants can be a suitable alternative. Carbamazepine is the drug of choice although it is less effective in the author's experience than tricyclics. Capsaicin cream has recently become available for treatment of painful peripheral neuropathy. It is applied twice daily to the skin and leads to depletion of substance P from nerve terminals. It has been effective in reducing burning pains in controlled trials,[18] although some patients find it too uncomfortable to use because of local skin irritation.

Occasionally neuropathic pain can become very severe, often in the context of sudden improvement in diabetic control, as is illustrated in the following case.

167

Case Study 28

A 21-year-old man was admitted for further assessment and treatment of severe pain in both feet. He had had type 1 diabetes since the age of 8 years, and his diabetic control had been consistently poor with HBA_{1c} results ranging between 9 and 13% over many years. Five months earlier he had been persuaded to switch from two to four injections of insulin daily, and he had received considerable input from the local diabetes specialist nurse. As a result his HBA_{1c} fell from 12.6 to 6%. Foot pains had started four weeks previously. He described an intense burning pain in a stocking distribution with shooting pains in both feet. His sleep was severely disrupted, he had lost his appetite, and his weight had fallen by 6 kg. Simple analgesics had been unhelpful, and he had only managed to achieve some relief by immersing his feet in cold water.

On examination his feet were hyperaemic, with excoriation of the skin from repeated immersion in water. He had normal peripheral circulation. He had no evidence of diabetic nephropathy but there was moderate background retinopathy on fundal examination.

He was treated with increasing doses of amitryptilene and carbamazepine over a week with little improvement. Simple analgesia was inadequate for acute pain control and he required regular morphine elixir with daily doses between 40 and 80 mg. He was transferred to long-acting morphine tablets, which made the pain tolerable. During his admission he ran near normal blood glucose levels and he was advised to lower his insulin doses to relax his overall level of glycaemic control. He was discharged two weeks later on morphine, amitryptilene, and carbamazepine. Over the subsequent six months his pain settled, and it was possible to tail off all his medication. He regained his weight and maintained much improved diabetic control.

This condition is termed acute painful neuropathy and can occur at any age and with any type of diabetes. The link with improved glycaemic control has been described in previous reports, although it is not known if the relationship is causal. This case report is typical in the severity of pain which may only respond to high doses of opiate. It is usually self-limiting after 9–18 months, and patients should be strongly reassured that their symptoms will eventually resolve.

Diabetic amyotrophy

Diabetic amyotrophy typically presents in middle-aged men, often with newly diagnosed or biochemically mild diabetes, with severe thigh pain associated with weakness and wasting of the quadriceps muscle group.[19] It can also occur in type 1 diabetes. The pain is continuous and usually described as an intense burning which is often so severe that it prevents sleep. Weakness can prevent the patient from attempting stairs. Both legs can be involved in up to 50% of cases, with the second leg usually becoming affected within one or two months of the first.[20] Wasting of the quadriceps is typical and the knee jerk is absent. Patients often lose a significant amount of weight during the acute episode.

The differential diagnosis includes lesions of the nerve roots, spinal cord, or cauda equina. In a typical presentation, a lumbar spine X-ray is probably all that is required but other investigations, including MR scanning, can be indicated to exclude spinal lesions if there are unusual features. The natural history is for the pain to resolve over an average of three months and muscle strength within one year. Treatment of the acute symptoms is with reassurance, tricyclic antidepressants, and analgesics for pain, and trying to improve diabetic control. Patients with type 2 diabetes are often put on insulin, although there is no evidence to suggest that recovery is affected by this. Anecdotally, some patients do feel better on insulin, and it may counter the weight loss.

Truncal radiculopathies

The usual presenting symptoms are of sudden onset of pain and dysaesthesia affecting the trunk, usually on one side. In the early stages it can be mistaken for herpes zoster infection before the appearance of the rash. Because of the location and distribution of the nerves, the differential diagnosis can include gallbladder disease, ischaemic heart disease, pleurisy, and musculoskeletal pain. As with other neuropathic pains in diabetes, it is often worse at night. Recovery usually occurs in six months or less.

Pressure neuropathies

The peripheral nerves are vulnerable to pressure damage, and carpal tunnel syndrome, foot drop, and Bell's palsy are all said to be more common than in non-diabetic subjects. Carpal tunnel syndrome presents with paraesthesia and numbness in the distribution of the median nerve. Pain often radiates to the elbow and is worse at night. Abduction of the thumb is weak and there may be wasting of the thenar eminence. Treatment is by surgical decompression of the median nerve at the wrist, although it is important to exclude hypothyroidism and acromegaly before proceeding to surgery.

Autonomic neuropathy

Autonomic neuropathy results from damage to the parasympathetic and sympathetic nerves, and usually occurs in patients who also have significant peripheral neuropathy. It can rarely cause a number of disabling symptoms. The main clinical features include diarrhoea, vomiting, postural hypotension, impotence, and gustatory sweating.

Diarrhoea is typically severe and disabling, and characteristically nocturnal. It often causes faecal incontinence. Intermittent periods of normal bowel function occur, that may last for weeks or months. Weight loss is unusual. The diagnosis is based on confirmation of autonomic neuropathy with cardiovascular autonomic function tests, and by exclusion of other causes of diarrhoea. It is important to exclude coeliac disease, which is more common in type 1 diabetes, and inflammatory or neoplastic bowel disease. Bacterial overgrowth can occur and may produce an abnormal hydrogen breath test (Chapter 6).

Treatment should include antidiarrhoeal agents, such as codeine phosphate or loperamide, sometimes in combination, tetracycline for bacterial overgrowth, as well as clonidine which may improve absorption of fluid from the intestine.

Gastric emptying is often delayed in diabetes, but it rarely causes clinical problems. Presentation is with intermittent vomiting, and a gastric splash on examination may provide a clinical clue. Structural causes of delayed gastric emptying must be excluded by endoscopy, and autonomic neuropathy confirmed. Treatment is with prokinetic drugs such as metoclopramide or cisapride. Short-term intravenous erythromycin improves gastric emptying by a direct action on motilin receptors in the gastrointestinal tract, but longer term oral therapy has proved less effective. Rarely parenteral nutrition is necessary.

Symptomatic postural hypotension is a rare feature of autonomic neuropathy, which may present with episodes of light-headedness or even syncope. Systolic blood pressure falls on standing by more than 30 mmHg. The diagnosis is confirmed by checking lying and standing blood pressures. Standing pressure should be measured after two minutes to allow time for blood pressure to fall. Diuretics and hypotensive drugs can exacerbate clinical symptoms. Occasionally, effective treatment of supine hypertension can be limited by postural hypotension. Patients should be advised to get up slowly, and drugs that exacerbate symptoms should be avoided. Fludrocortisone (50–100 µg o.d.) can be tried to promote salt and water retention, it usually causes oedema before it helps the dizziness.

References

1 Young MJ, Boulton AJM, MacLeod AFD, Williams DDR, Sonksen PH. A multicentre study of the prevalence of diabetic peripheral neuropathy in the United Kingdom. Hospital clinic population. *Diabetologia* 1993;**36**:150–4.

2 Pirart J. Diabetes mellitus and its degenerative complications. A prospective study of 4000 patients observed. *Diabetes Care* 1978;**1**: 168–88, 252–63.

3 Delbridge L, Le Quesne LP. Leg support for the post-operative protection of the heel in patients with diabetes. *Br J Surg* 1985;**72**:87.

4 Siitonen OI, Niskanen LK, Laasko LK, Siitonen JT, Pyorala K. Lower extremity amputation in diabetic and non-diabetic patients: a population-based study in eastern Finland. *Diabetes Care* 1993;**16**: 16–20.

5 Wagner FW. Algorithms of diabetic foot care. In: Levin ME, O'Neil LW, eds. *The diabetic foot*, 2nd edn. St Louis: Mosby Yearbook, 1983: 291–302.

6 Burden AC, Jones GR, Jones R, Blandford RL. Use of the "Scotchcast boot" in treating diabetic foot ulcers. *Br Med J* 1983;**286**:1555–7.

7 Gentry LO. Diagnosis and management of the diabetic foot ulcer. *J Antimicrob Chemother* 1993;**32**:77–89.

8 Venkatesan P, Lawn S, Macfarlare RM *et al.* Conservative management of osteomyelitis in the foot of diabetic patients. *Diabetic Med* 1997;**14**: 487–90.

9 Stonebridge PA, Murie JA. Infrainguinal revascularisation in the diabetic patient. *Br J Surg* 1993;**80**:1237–41.

10 Sutton G, Wolfe J. Distal revascularisation and the diabetic foot. *Practical Diabetes* 1994;**11**:95–6.

11 Mamode N, Scott RN, McLaughlin SC, McLelland A, Pollock JG. Perioperative myocardial infarction in peripheral vascular surgery. *Br Med J* 1996;**312**:1396–7.

12 Dormandly J. Use of the prostacyclin analogue iloprost in the treatment of patients with critical limb ischaemia. *Therapie* 1991;**46**:319–22.

13 Gentzkow GD, Iwasaki SD, Hershon KS *et al.* Use of dermagraft, a cultured human dermis, to treat diabetic foot ulcers. *Diabetes Care* 1996;**19**:350–4.

14 Selby PL, Young MJ, Boulton AJM. Bisphosphonates: A new treatment for diabetic Charcot neuroarthropathy? *Diabetic Med* 1994;**11**:28–31.

15 Most RS, Sinnock P. The epidemiology of lower extremity amputation in diabetic individuals. *Diabetes Care* 1983;**6**:87–91.

16 Deerochanawong C, Home PD, Alberti KGMM. A survey of lower limb amputation in diabetic patients. *Diabetic Med* 1992;**9**:942–6.

17 Young RJ. Pain relief in diabetic neuropathy: the effectiveness of imipramine and related drugs. *Diabetic Med* 1985;**2**:363–6.

18 Capsaicin Study Group. Treatment of painful diabetic neuropathy with topical capsaicin. A multicentre, double blind, vehicle-controlled study. *Ann Intern Med* 1991;**151**:2225–9.

19 Coppack S, Watkins PJ. The natural history of femoral neuropathy. *Q J Med* 1991;**79**:307–13.

20 Donaghy M. Diabetic proximal neuropathy: Therapy and prognosis. *Q J Med* 1991;**79**:287–8.

9 Diabetes and the eye

Despite the availability of effective treatment for over 20 years, diabetic retinopathy remains the commonest cause of blindness in people of working age (Table 9.1). The continued high incidence of visual loss partly reflects the increasing prevalence of diabetes but inadequate screening and delayed referral also play a part. The importance of effective screening for diabetic retinopathy was brought into sharp focus by the settlement of an action against a UK health authority for £225 000 in 1992, for a failure to screen and appropriately refer a woman with type 2 diabetes who had attended a hospital diabetes clinic for 12 years.[1]

In this chapter the clinical features of diabetic retinopathy are described, together with the recommended referral guidelines for different degrees of severity and the appropriate screening intervals for patients with diabetes. Other eye problems which occur more commonly in diabetes are also described.

Epidemiology

The epidemiology has been well documented in prospective trials. The population-based Wisconsin Epidemiologic Study of Diabetic Retinopathy (WESDR) used ophthalmoscopy and photographs to document the incidence and prevalence of

Table 9.1   Causes of avoidable blindness in people of working age in England and Wales, 1990–1991[2]

Registration	Partial sight		Blindness	
	Cases	(%)	Cases	(%)
Diabetic retinopathy	229	(36.6)	234	(49.2)
Glaucoma	111	(17.7)	89	(18.7)
Cataracts	110	(17.7)	42	(8.8)
Retinal detachments and defects	41	(6.5)	27	(5.7)
Injuries	30	(4.8)	23	(4.8)
Others	105	(16.7)	61	(12.8)

retinopathy over a 10-year period.[3] Three groups of patients were identified: young patients taking insulin who were diagnosed at <30 years of age, older patients diagnosed ⩾30 years who were taking diet and tablets, and finally an older group whose diabetes was diagnosed at >30 years of age and who were treated with insulin.

Overall, the prevalence of retinopathy increased with disease duration in all groups, but important differences were seen between patients with type 1, type 2, and the group of older patients taking insulin who were a mix of type 1 and 2 diabetes.

Type 1 diabetes

Retinopathy was not found at diagnosis of type 1 diabetes, and was uncommon during the first few years, with 17% of patients having minor retinopathy five years after diagnosis. Beyond that, background retinopathy, characterised by microaneurysms, blot haemorrhages, and hard exudates (Figure 9.1) became more

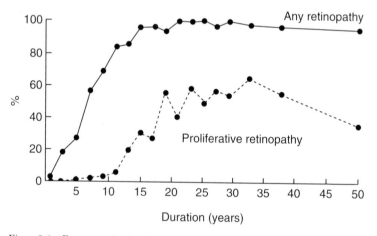

Figure 9.1 Frequency of retinopathy or proliferative retinopathy by duration of diabetes in years.

common; at 10 years, approximately 50%; and at 20 years nearly all had background retinopathy.[4]

Proliferative retinopathy, characterised by sight-threatening retinal neovascularisation, was not seen before five years after diagnosis, but the prevalence increased to 26% within 15 years, and 50% within 20 years after diagnosis.

Several factors have been associated with an increased risk of developing diabetic retinopathy (Box 9.1)

Box 9.1 Established factors associated with a higher risk of diabetic retinopathy

- Duration of diabetes
- Poor glycaemic control
- Hypertension
- Proteinuria
- Male sex

Type 2 diabetes

In the Wisconsin study, of those diagnosed >30 years of age, 20% had background retinopathy at diagnosis.[5] This reflects the "preclinical" phase of diabetes, often lasting for several years. After 15 years about half those treated with diet and tablets and 80% of insulin-treated patients had retinopathy (Figure 9.2). Proliferative retinopathy was not as common in older patients, occurring in 20–25% after 20 years' disease duration. Background and proliferative retinopathy were more common in older patients taking insulin, probably because of their longer disease duration.

Diabetic maculopathy, characterised by leakage of fluid from microaneurysms or dilated capillaries in the macular region of the retina, was more common in older patients on insulin compared to those on diet and tablets, with a prevalence approaching 25% after 20 years of diabetes.

Physical signs in diabetic retinopathy

Outside specialist ophthalmic practice, diabetic retinopathy is best diagnosed by examination of the retina, through dilated pupils, with a direct ophthalmoscope. The following features may be seen:

- *Microaneurysms* (also known as "dots"). These are caused by saccular outpouchings of retinal capillaries and are usually the

175

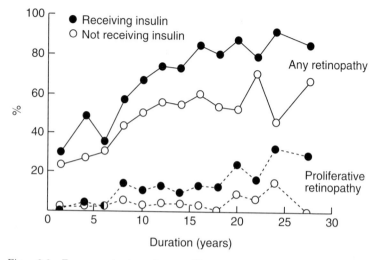

Figure 9.2 Frequency of retinopathy or proliferative retinopathy by duration of insulin-taking and non-insulin-taking persons.

first detectable signs of retinopathy. The number and distribution of microaneurysms varies with time, but they tend to occur most commonly at the pole of the eye and temporal to the macula.

- *Intraretinal haemorrhages.* The shape of an intraretinal haemorrhage depends on its depth in the retinal nerve fibre layer. Dot and blot haemorrhages are located deep in the retina whereas flame-shaped haemorrhages are more superficial and are often associated with systemic hypertension.
- *Hard exudates.* These are waxy white lipoprotein deposits resulting from capillary leakage, a feature of diabetic microvascular disease. They appear as white dots that often coalesce into clusters, linear streaks near the fovea, and large "circinate" rings.
- *Macular oedema.* Oedema results from abnormally permeable retinal vessels which allow leakage of plasma contents into retinal nerve fibres. Oedema fluid accumulates in the macular region (the retinal area two disc diameters around the fovea) and causes gradual visual loss. It can be very difficult to detect with direct ophthalmoscopy, and the only clue to diagnosis may be a gradual reduction in visual acuity, not improved by spectacles or a pinhole.

- *Cottonwool spots* (retinal infarcts). These appear as indistinct round or oval lesions in the nerve fibre layer. They are usually first seen in the nasal retina and the mid-peripheral retina around the vascular arcades. Five or more cottonwool spots in a fundus is associated with a two-fold increased risk of proliferative retinopathy over the following year.
- *Intravascular microvascular abnormalities (IRMA)*. These are abnormally shaped capillaries, often with the appearance of a lacy network developing within the retina. They are a sign of progressive ischaemia and carry a high risk of future new vessel formation.
- *Venous changes*. These are characterised by beading, when the major veins have the appearance of "a string of sausages" and venous loops. Both are signs of severe retinal ischaemia and predict a four-fold increased risk of new vessels within one year.
- *Arteriolar changes*. These occur with narrow tortuous vessels and are also a sign of severe ischaemia. Occasionally an arteriolar branch will occlude completely, leaving a white line.
- *New vessels*. These cardinal features of proliferative retinopathy develop in response to growth factors from the ischaemic retina. New vessels grow from retinal veins and extend through the internal limiting membrane of the retina, to lie between this and the vitreous surface. They may therefore be intraretinal, flat on the retinal surface, or raised. The optic disc is most commonly affected (termed new vessels disc, NVD), but they may also occur in the mid-periphery of the retina (termed new vessels elsewhere, NVE). In addition, other features of severe ischaemia are usually present, including venous changes, cottonwool spots, and IRMA. New vessels on the iris, termed rubeosis, are a sign of severe ischaemia and lead to the development of secondary neovascular glaucoma by obstruction of the drainage channels of the aqueous.
- *Preretinal haemorrhages*. These flat-topped haemorrhages occur as a result of bleeding from new vessels. They are an important sign of new vessels, even though the haemorrhage may obscure them.
- *Vitreous haemorrhage*. This is the most severe consequence of neovascularisation and the commonest cause of acute visual loss in patients with diabetes. A dense vitreous haemorrhage appears as a grey opacity on direct fundoscopy, and it is often impossible to see the fundus or identify the neovascular complex responsible

177

for the bleeding. Vitreous haemorrhage can persist for weeks or years, and often prevents laser photocoagulation. A persistent vitreous haemorrhage is an indication for vitrectomy.

- *Gliosis.* This refers to the presence of white scar tissue which forms together with neovascular elements. The gliotic scars are often seen around the vascular arcades, where they contract and may give rise to traction retinal detachment.

Classification of diabetic retinopathy

It is clinically useful to classify retinopathy into sight- and non-sight-threatening categories, because this helps to define a management plan, and determines whether referral for ophthalmological opinion is necessary and, if so, how urgently.

Sight-threatening retinopathy can be defined as asymptomatic retinopathy likely to cause visual loss within the foreseeable future (Box 9.2).

Preproliferative and proliferative retinopathy do not affect visual acuity, unless haemorrhage occurs, when there may be sudden visual loss. Patients may describe a "curtain coming down in one eye" or a "cobweb" in their field of vision. In contrast, maculopathy typically causes a gradual deterioration in vision over months or years, and this is the main reason for including an assessment of visual acuity in the screening procedure. Lesser degrees of background retinopathy are symptomless and do not require treatment.

Screening for diabetic retinopathy

Since retinopathy is symptomless until complications develop, regular screening should be an essential part of the diabetic management plan (Table 9.2). Recommended intervals for screening are shown in the table. Sight-threatening retinopathy is unlikely to develop during the first 10 years after diagnosis of type 1 diabetes, and this is reflected in the recommended screening interval. However, if retinopathy is seen before 10 years, annual screening should be adopted as for type 2 diabetes. The screening interval should be shortened to every three to six months in all patients where retinopathy is found.

Box 9.2 Features of sight-threatening retinopathy that require ophthalmic referral

Sight-threatening maculopathy
- Foveal oedema
- Hard exudates within one disc diameter of the fovea
- Macular oedema within two disc diameters of the fovea
- Multiple exudates above and below the fovea
- Multiple microaneurysms and haemorrhages within the temporal arcades

Preproliferative retinopathy
- Venous beading and/or venous loops
- Arteriolar thinning and/or white lines
- IRMA
- Multiple cottonwool spots (more than five in one hemifield)
- Multiple haemorrhages in the mid-peripheral veins

Proliferative retinopathy
- New vessels on the optic disc, or in the retinal mid-periphery near vascular arcades

Advanced diabetic eye disease
- Preretinal haemorrhage or vitreous haemorrhage
- Macular distortion
- Traction retinal detachment
- Rubeosis iridis
- Neovascular glaucoma

Annual retinal examination is essential in all patients with type 2 diabetes from diagnosis. In the United Kingdom Prospective Diabetes Study, patients without retinopathy had a 1% chance of needing laser treatment after six years compared with a 30% chance in those with moderate background retinopathy at initial retinal examination.[6]

A comprehensive clerking of a patient with diabetes should always include details of when their eyes were last examined *through dilated pupils* and who did it. Arrangements should be made for an eye examination to be performed if appropriate screening has not been done. It should be emphasised that this applies to *newly diagnosed* type 2 diabetes patients who occasionally present with sight-threatening retinopathy as is shown in the case study below.

Table 9.2 Recommended screening intervals of the European Retinopathy Working Party[7]

Diabetes	At diagnosis	Screening intervals		Increased frequency (3–6 monthly)
		0–10 years	>10 years	
Type 1	Yes	Every 2 years	Annually	Established retinopathy Pregnancy Diabetic nephropathy
Type 2	Yes	Annually	Annually	Established retinopathy Nephropathy

Case Study 29

A 54-year-old man was referred to the hospital diabetes clinic for assessment of recently diagnosed type 2 diabetes. He had seen his GP with recurrent balanitis; diabetes had been confirmed with blood glucose measurements. He had no visual symptoms. Examination revealed visual acuities of 6/6 in both eyes, but there was florid proliferative retinopathy (Figure 9.3) of both optic discs. He was also noted to have sensory neuropathy and Albustix-positive proteinuria. He was referred urgently to the ophthalmology department and received extensive laser photocoagulation the following week.

Review of his medical notes showed a record of a urine sample taken during an appointment in a different clinic 10 years previously which contained + + glucose, but which had been overlooked.

The case illustrates that severe sight-threatening retinopathy can be a feature of *apparently* newly diagnosed diabetes. It has been estimated that patients presenting with retinopathy have had undiagnosed diabetes for between four and six years (Figure 9.4).[8] The record of glycosuria 10 years previously in this case suggests that undiagnosed diabetes may run a much longer course in some patients.

How to screen for diabetic retinopathy (Box 9.3)

Vision

A diabetic eye check should begin with an assessment of visual acuity. This is tested using a well-illuminated Snellen chart, with

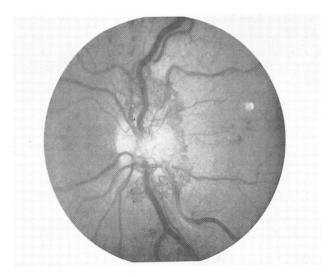

Figure 9.3   Fundus.

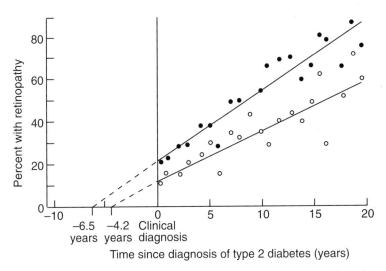

Figure 9.4   Prevalence of any retinopathy according to years since clinical diagnosis of type 2 diabetes among patients in Southern Wisconsin (●) and in rural Western Australia (○). Solid lines, data fitted by weighted linear regression. Lines are extrapolated to indicate the time at which onset of observable retinopathy is estimated to have occurred. $R^2 = 0.89$ and 0.80 for Wisconsin and Australia, respectively.

the patient 6 metres away. Visual acuity is assessed by asking the patient to read the smallest letters on the Snellen chart that they are able to. This is expressed as 6 over the corresponding size of letter which the patient can read. So, for example, a patient who can only see size 18 letters has an acuity of 6/18 meaning they can see letters at 6 metres, which a person with normal eyesight should be able to see at 18 metres. Failure to see one or two letters on a line should be recorded as, for example, 6/12 (−2) if 2 letters were incorrectly read. Normal vision is 6/6 or better. If the largest letter cannot be seen, the vision is worse than 6/60. The patient should be asked if they can count fingers (CF), assess hand movements (HM) or perceive light (PL).

Box 9.3 Summary of screening procedure diabetic eye complications[7]

- Identification and collection of clinical data
- Onset of visual symptoms
- History of glaucoma
- Measurement of visual acuity unaided and, if necessary, with glasses and/or pinhole
- Pupil dilatation with an appropriate mydriatic
- Lens examination for cataract with a + 10 lens in ophthalmoscopy
- Fundus examination

Spectacles should be worn if the patient usually wears them for distance vision. If a patient has fogotten spectacles or acuity is worse than 6/9 in either eye, the acuity should be repeated with the patient looking through a pinhole; an improvement suggests a refractive problem, whereas no improvement suggests a lens opacity or macular problem. Once acuity has been recorded, mydriatic drops should be instilled to dilate the pupils. A variety of drugs can be used, but 0.5 or 1% tropicamide drops are ideal because they work within 20–30 minutes and usually last for two to three hours. Other agents such as cyclopentolate or phenylephrine have a longer duration of action. The risk of precipitating acute open angle glaucoma with tropicamide is extremely small and it can be argued that, even if this does occur, it will bring a treatable eye condition to medical attention.

After mydriasis the fundus should be examined. Two techniques can be used; direct ophthalmoscopy or a fundal camera with Polaroid, 35 mm film, or digital computer imaging.

Direct fundoscopy

A systematic approach in eye examination is important. The anterior chamber and lens should be examined first by looking for the "red reflex" in each eye from about 30 cm with a +10 lens and noting the presence of any cataract. The next landmark, as the ophthalmoscope is brought close to the patient's eye, is the optic disc. Because new vessels often grow out towards the vitreous rather than over the retina, it is usually necessary to "rack" through the lenses when the disc is being examined to get a three-dimensional image. Once the disc has been carefully examined, the major vascular arcades should be followed to the peripheral retina in each of the quadrants, their calibre and appearance noted, together with associated retinal appearances of haemorrhages and exudates. Examine the macula by asking the patient to look directly into the light; then assess the retina temporal to the macula by asking the patient to look towards the side you are examining. This systematic approach allows all areas of the fundus to be examined, and the results can be recorded on a fundal diagram.

As with all clinical skills, ophthalmoscopy requires training and practice. The sensitivity of "unselected" hospital doctors is of the order of 30–40% in identifying sight-threatening retinopathy or, put another way, six or seven cases out of 10 can be missed. Sensitivity improves with training and experience, and most studies suggest a sensitivity of about 70% for experienced diabetologists. Specificity, the ability to recognise normal appearances, is better and approaches 90% in most studies.

Fundal cameras

Fundal cameras offer an alternative approach to fundal examination and are available in some hospitals; provided patients are examined after mydriasis, these cameras achieve similar sensitivity and specificity as direct ophthalmoscopy by an experienced diabetologist. Optimal performance is obtained when 35 mm rather than Polaroid film is used, and when at least two retinal photographs, one centred on the fovea and one on the disc, are taken. Sensitivity increases with four- or seven-field retinal photography, but these are generally used only for research purposes. For a variety of reasons up to 15% of photographs are not of sufficient quality for accurate assessment; this figure rises in the over-50s, because mydriasis is less effective and because of a higher prevalence of cataract.

183

Retinal cameras are generally better at detecting maculopathy and macular oedema but direct ophthalmoscopy is more sensitive at identifying new vessels, because it is easier to obtain a three-dimensional assessment. Some advocate using both screening modalities to obtain as accurate a screening method as possible.[9]

Referral for identified retinopathy

The European Retinopathy Working Party suggestions for referral guidelines to a specialist ophthalmologist are included in Box 9.4.

In general it is better to err on the side of caution, since it is relatively easy for an ophthalmologist to assess a patient and give reassurance if there is no serious problem.

Treatment

Photocoagulation

Laser photocoagulation is the treatment of choice for proliferative retinopathy and maculopathy. In proliferative retinopathy between 1500 and 3000 laser burns are applied around the temporal arcades (avoiding the macular region) and to the peripheral retina temporal to the macula. Destruction of the peripheral retina reduces the retinal oxygen demand and hence the release of growth factors responsible for neovascularisation. Peripheral new vessels are also treated with laser photocoagulation, although this may be confined to a sector of the retina rather than being pan-retinal.

Pan-retinal photocoagulation is a highly effective treatment, which reduced the risk of vitreous haemorrhage, advanced diabetic eye disease, and severe visual loss in the Early Treatment Diabetic Retinopathy Study (ETDRS) by over 50%.[10] It is important to note, however, that up to 25% of those treated still develop severe visual loss five years after treatment. Data from the ETDRS also support laser treatment for severe preproliferative retinopathy, which can reduce the risk of progression to severe visual loss by about 50%.

Exudative maculopathy with circinate rings of hard exudates in the macular region requires a different approach. Grid laser applied to the central area of a circinate ring with the objective of reducing capillary leakage can prevent further visual deterioration in about

184

Box 9.4 ERWP referral guidelines

Immediate	Same day Telephone referral	• *Proliferative retinopathy* • disc new vessels or new vessels elsewhere • pre-retinal haemorrhage • *Advanced diabetic eye disease* • vitreous haemorrhage • recent retinal detachment • fibrous tissue • rubeosis iridis
Soon	Letter	• *Preproliferative retinopathy* • venous irregularities (beading, loops) • multiple haemorrhages, within vascular arcades • multiple cottonwool spots • IRMA • *Maculopathy* • reduced acuity not corrected by pinhole (possible macula oedema) • haemorrhages/exudates within one disc diameter of the fovea
Routine	Letter	• *Non-proliferative retinopathy without macular involvement* • circinate or plaque hard exudates within major temporal vascular arcades • any abnormality the observer cannot interpret

60% of patients, although some continue to deteriorate despite apparently effective laser treatment.[11] Ischaemic maculopathy, characterised by non-perfusion of the perifoveal capillary arcades, does not respond to photocoagulation. Fluorescein angiography may be useful to determine the specific type of maculopathy and whether photocoagulation is likely to be beneficial.

Laser treatment is usually performed as an outpatient procedure. A lens is applied to the cornea after instillation of local anaesthetic drops, and laser burns are applied with the patient and operator seated at a slit lamp. Initial pan-retinal photocoagulation can

185

usually be completed in three or four "sittings", and grid laser usually requires only one or two. Occasionally a patient cannot tolerate photocoagulation or is unable to cooperate and requires admission for a short general anaesthetic to allow the treatment to be applied. Diabetes management during day-case procedures is discussed in Chapter 5.

Vitrectomy

Vitrectomy is indicated for persistent vitreous haemorrhage and recent retinal detachment. The procedure involves removal of the cloudy vitreous in stages with a mechanical cutter and simultaneous replacement with saline. Dissection of fibrous membranes is also possible to reduce traction on the retina and lessen the risk of future retinal detachment. It is possible to give laser photocoagulation during the procedure to complete pan-retinal treatment and to re-apply detached retina. Overall about 60–70% of patients have a good result from vitreoretinal surgery.[12]

"At-risk patients"

Improved glycaemic control

Studies looking at the effect of intensified diabetic control have consistently found that retinopathy deteriorates in the first year after control is improved. This is clinically apparent as an increase in the number of retinal infarcts (cottonwool spots) and may occasionally require photocoagulation. The reasons are unclear, but it may reflect an acute fall in retinal blood flow and increased ischaemia. It should not deter attempts to improve control, since the long-term outcome is much better than if poor control persists. The likelihood of deterioration is related to the initial severity of the retinopathy; those with moderate background retinopathy or worse should be reviewed more frequently, possibly every four to six months, if glycaemic control needs to be tightened.

Pregnancy

Retinopathy can deteriorate during pregnancy, possibly as a result of the improved glycaemic control that is usually achieved. Ideally patients should have a full retinal examination before conception. Patients with proliferative retinopathy require urgent referral for photocoagulation and should ideally delay pregnancy. Women with background retinopathy should be re-examined each trimester through dilated pupils and, if there are signs of progressive ischaemia, referral for possible laser photocoagulation should be considered. Retinopathy at conception and hypertension are both significant predictors of the chances of its progression during pregnancy.

Nephropathy

Patients with nephropathy usually have significant retinopathy. This association is clinically "robust", and finding a patient with renal impairment who does not have retinopathy should raise the possibility of non-diabetic renal disease. Exceptions to this dogma include Asians who are more likely to develop nephropathy than Caucasians (Chapter 10).

As renal function declines, retinopathy usually worsens and, in some patients with nephrotic range proteinuria, severe macular oedema may develop which is difficult to treat. Retinal examination should be performed every four to six months in patients with nephropathy to identify treatable retinopathy.

Other ocular problems

Cataract

Cataracts (Figure 9.5) develop earlier and progress more rapidly in diabetic subjects. In the Wisconsin study 59% of patients aged 30–54 years had cataracts compared with 12% of non-diabetic controls.[5] Cataracts develop earlier in diabetes because hyperglycaemia causes non-enzymatic glycation of lens proteins. Rarely the lens may opacify over a few days or even overnight in young patients with recently diagnosed type 1 diabetes, causing a "snowflake" cataract, which may clear spontaneously but may require extraction. The more typical appearance is of cortical cataracts which produce a spokewheel appearance when examined with the ophthalmoscope. Cortical cataracts gradually progress with central lens opacification, leading to loss of visual acuity. Once the whole lens becomes opaque the term "mature cataract" is used and this in time may progress to a hypermature cataract, in which the capsule becomes permeable to lens proteins or fluid. This may cause an inflammatory glaucoma which requires early cataract extraction.

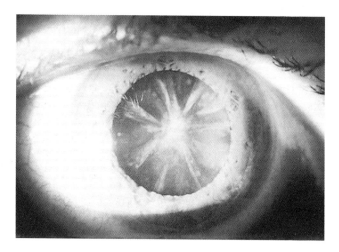

Figure 9.5   Cataract.

A posterior subcapsular cataract consists of recently formed opaque lens fibres lying in front of the posterior capsule that tend to cause troublesome visual loss at an early stage because of their central position.

Cataract surgery is commonly undertaken in patients with diabetes, usually because of deteriorating vision sufficiently severe to interfere with quality of life. A second important indication for surgery is to allow assessment or treatment of the retinopathy to continue, where this has been rendered impossible by the cataract. Surgery can usually be carried out under local anaesthetic as a day case and, since it causes only minor metabolic disturbance, management of hyperglycaemia during the procedure is usually straightforward. Diabetes management guidelines for day case surgery are described in Chapter 5.

It is important to assess whether a cataract is sufficient to account for the patient's difficulties. A mild cataract with poor acuity may suggest coexistent retinal pathology that may need treatment. The decision to undertake cataract surgery in a diabetic subject has to be carefully weighed, since the postoperative period may be associated with significant morbidity particularly affecting the retina. Cataract extraction may result in a worsening of retinopathy, particularly maculopathy, especially in those with more severe retinal disease prior to surgery.[13]

Sudden visual loss

Vitreous haemorrhage is the commonest cause of sudden visual loss in diabetes, but other conditions should be considered. Many are related to vascular disease and therefore occur more commonly, but not exclusively, in patients with diabetes. In most cases nothing can be done to restore vision, but it is important to identify retinal detachment where timely intervention can restore vision and prevent anterior ischaemic optic neuropathy, which may be related to temporal arteritis when treatment with steroids should protect the other eye. The key to successful diagnosis lies in the history and appearance of the fundus.

Anterior ischaemic optic neuropathy (AION)

The blood supply to the optic disc is cut off, causing infarction. Typically, this presents as sudden onset of a central scotoma with preservation of peripheral vision. Fundal examination shows a swollen pale optic disc with flame-shaped haemorrhages. It occurs in young patients with type 1 diabetes, and is termed the optic neuropathy of juvenile diabetes. The long-term prognosis is good with gradual improvement in vision occurring over two to three months.

Central retinal artery occlusion

This presents as a sudden painless loss of vision down to hand movement or perception of light only. It is due to retinal artery thrombosis, or emboli from the heart or carotid vessels, typically in patients >60 years of age. There may be a history of amaurosis fugax—transient uniocular visual loss owing to platelet emboli from the ipsilateral carotid artery. In the early stages fundal appearances are often normal, although pallor with threadlike arterioles and a "cherry red spot" over the fovea are the classically described features. The cherry red spot is the view of the underlying choroid vessels, the remainder of which are obscured by the oedematous and infarcted retina. Branch retinal artery occlusions occur and are also related to vascular emboli, which can sometimes be seen within a vessel as a white "glistening" object, usually at a vessel bifurcation. Visual field loss in the affected retina is permanent although the visual prognosis for the eye as a whole is good if the macula is spared.

A patient with diabetes presenting with a central or branch retinal artery occlusion should be carefully evaluated for hypertension, hyperlipidaemia, carotid arterial disease, cardiac arrhythmias, and murmurs. Appropriate treatment of identified vascular risk factors should reduce the chances of other events occurring.

An important differential diagnosis of central retinal artery occlusion is temporal arteritis, and clinical features, such as temporal headache and jaw claudication, and systemic symptoms, including malaise and weight loss, should always be sought, together with a raised ESR usually >80 mm/h. If the diagnosis seems likely, high-dose steroids (prednisolone 60–100 mg/day) should be started to protect the other eye. Blood glucose will inevitably rise after two to three days, and this will require careful monitoring and adjustment of treatment. It is often necessary to switch patients on oral hypoglycaemic drugs to insulin, and regular review of the patient by the diabetes team is an important part of management (Chapter 2).

Central retinal vein occlusion

This is associated with diabetes, hypertension, smoking, glaucoma, and occasionally with hyperviscosity states. Vision is moderately or severely affected and retinal examination shows disc oedema with widespread haemorrhages in all quadrants and occasional cottonwool spots. Branch vein or hemiretinal vein occlusions also occur, in which symptoms are less marked and the fundal abnormalities restricted to one quadrant. There is no immediate treatment but patients require regular ophthalmic review because of the risk of retinal ischaemia with neovascularisation. Laser photocoagulation can help to prevent secondary glaucoma, pain, and possibly loss of the eye.

The prognosis for vision is variable, but some patients experience a return of useful vision. In about 10% the other eye suffers a similar fate at a later stage.

Retinal detachment

This usually presents as flashes and floaters and patients may also describe a grey curtain in the periphery of their vision. Visual field loss corresponds to the area of detachment which may include the macular area. These symptoms require urgent (same day) referral since re-attachment of the retina using cryotherapy or laser therapy may restore vision, but only if it is undertaken within a day or so of the detachment.

Neovascular glaucoma

This occurs as a complication of rubeosis iridis and severe ischaemic retinopathy. It causes acute painful visual loss as a result of increased intraocular pressure and corneal oedema. Treatment is difficult, and occasionally enucleation may be the only effective treatment for an eye which is blind and intractably painful.

Ocular palsies

These usually affect the third or sixth nerve and are relatively common in type 2 diabetes. The typical presentation is with sudden onset of painless diplopia, which gradually resolves over weeks or months. With a third nerve palsy there is usually sparing of the pupillary reflex and this helps to distinguish between a third nerve palsy caused by a posterior communicating artery aneurysm in which the pupil is usually fixed and dilated. It is usually necessary to prescribe prisms to spectacles if they are worn, or to occlude the affected eye in order to deal with the diplopia whilst the patient is awaiting recovery.

It is difficult to lay down rules as to whether patients with diabetes who present with a third nerve palsy require cranial imaging to exclude an intracerebral aneurysm, and each case must be judged on its merits. Where the presentation is classical, it is reasonable to await gradual improvement and resist the urge to order a cranial CT scan or arteriogram.

References

1 Brahams D. Medicine and the law. Eye monitoring in diabetes. *Lancet* 1992;**339**:863–4.

2 Evans J, Rooney C, Ashwood F, Dattani N, Wormald R. Blindness and partial sight in England and Wales: April 1990–March 1991. *Health Trends* 1996;**28**:5–12.

3 Klein R, Klein BEK, Moss SE, Cruickshanks KJ. The Wisconsin Epidemiologic Study of Diabetic Retinopathy XIV. Ten year incidence and progression of diabetic retinopathy. *Arch Ophthalmol* 1994;**112**: 1217–28.

4 Klein R, Klein BEK, Moss SE *et al*. The Wisconsin Epidemiologic Study of Diabetic Retinopathy II. Prevalence and risk of diabetic retinopathy when age at diagnosis is less than 30 years. *Arch Ophthalmol* 1984;**102**:520–6.

5 Klein R, Klein BEK, Moss SE *et al*. The Wisconsin Epidemiologic Study of Diabetic Retinopathy III. Prevalence and risk of diabetic retinopathy when age at diagnosis is 30 or more years. *Arch Ophthalmol* 1984;**102**:527–32.

6 Stratton IM, Matthews DR, Kohner E *et al*. Evaluating risk of progression to photocoagulation by retinal photography or direct ophthalmoscopy. *Diabetologia* 1997; **40** (Suppl 1): A17, Abstract 60.

7 European Retinopathy Working Party Report. A protocol for screening for diabetic retinopathy in Europe. *Diabetic Med* 1991;**8**:263–7.

8 Harris MI, Klein R, Welborn T, Knuiman MW. Onset of NIDDM occurs at least 4–7 years before clinical diagnosis. *Diabetes Care* 1992; **15**:815–19.

9 Ryder B. Screening for diabetic retinopathy; combined modalities seem to offer the best option. *Br Med J* 1995;**311**:207–8.

10 Early Treatment Diabetic Retinopathy Study Research Group. Photocoagulation treatment of proliferative diabetic retinopathy. Clinical application of DRS findings. DRS report number 8. *Ophthalmology* 1981;**88**:583–600.

11 Early Treatment Diabetic Retinopathy Study Research Group. Photocoagulation treatment for diabetic macular edema. ETDRS report number 1. *Ophthalmology* 1985;**103**:1796–806.

12 Early Treatment Diabetic Retinopathy Study Research Group. Pars planar vitrectomy in the early treatment diabetic retinopathy study. ETDRS study number 17. *Ophthalmology* 1992;**99**:1351–7.

13 Dowler JGF, Hykin PG, Lightman SL *et al*. Visual acuity following extracapsular cataract extraction in diabetes: a meta-analysis. *Eye* 1995;**9**:313–17.

10 Diabetic nephropathy and other renal emergencies in diabetes

Diabetic nephropathy is one of the commonest causes of end-stage renal failure and accounts for about one in three patients accepted for dialysis.[1] The natural history of diabetic nephropathy is one of progressive renal failure developing over many years, but patients sometimes need urgent admission for the treatment of fluid retention, hypertension, electrolyte imbalance, and the nephrotic syndrome. In addition, a number of other complications occur in diabetes, including renovascular disease and hyporeninaemic hypoaldosteronism, which can present as urgent management problems. Renal tract infections are discussed in Chapter 11.

In this chapter the natural history of diabetic nephropathy and its clinical management will be described and some of the problems of management discussed. Other renal complications associated with diabetes will also be discussed.

Natural history of diabetic nephropathy

In the UK, about 600 patients require dialysis owing to diabetic nephropathy each year and, as with most Western countries, this number is increasing. Patients with type 1 diabetes diagnosed <30 years of age are at greatest risk. As with all microvascular complications, the prevalence of nephropathy increases with disease duration but, after 30 years, and in marked contrast to retinopathy, only about 35% will have evidence of renal involvement, suggesting that there is a subpopulation of such patients who are susceptible to renal damage (see below). Glycaemic control is a strong predictor of progression to end-stage renal failure (ESRF). In a 35-year follow-up of 142 patients with type 1 diabetes attending the Joslin Diabetes Centre, ESRF developed in 36% of patients who were in the worst tertile of glycaemic control, but only 14.4 and 9.2% respectively in the middle and best tertiles.[2]

The risk of an individual patient with type 2 diabetes reaching ESRF is less than in those with type 1 but, because the former is more common, greater numbers of these patients are accepted for ESRF treatment each year in many countries.[3] The global epidemic of type 2 diabetes is likely to increase demand for renal dialysis services in the future.

Certain racial groups are at high risk of developing diabetic nephropathy. Studies in Leicestershire in the UK suggest that the relative risk of ESRF in people of Asian origin was 13.6 times greater than in Caucasians.[4] Patients of Afro-Caribbean origin also carry a significantly increased risk.[5]

Pathophysiology

Diabetic nephropathy is a disease of the renal microcirculation, resulting in progressive scarring of the capillaries in the glomerular tuft. Much more is known of how this damage occurs in type 1 than in type 2 diabetes.

Type 1 diabetes

- *Genetic factors*
  Only about 30–35% of patients will develop nephropathy, suggesting there is variation in individual susceptibility. Family studies suggest a genetic predisposition with a three-fold increased risk in first-degree relatives of a proband with nephropathy.[6] The gene or genes have not been identified.

- *Haemodynamic factors*
  The kidneys are often enlarged at diagnosis, mainly owing to increased glomerular size, and this is associated with an increased glomerular filtration rate. In susceptible subjects, hyperfiltration may contribute to haemodynamic changes, particularly raised glomerular filtration pressure, which predispose to glomerular damage.

- *Metabolic factors*
  Hyperglycaemia damages glomeruli in several ways:
  - non-enzymatic glycation alters the electrical charge of the basement membrane, within glomeruli, allowing leakage of negatively charged proteins such as albumin;
  - metabolic changes occur within mesangial cells leading to the abnormal accumulation of metabolites, such as sorbitol;
  - hyperglycaemia stimulates growth factors, causing expansion of mesangial tissues, an important histological feature of nephropathy.

Diabetic nephropathy results from widespread damage to glomeruli which leads to progressive inability of the kidneys to maintain normal filtration of the blood. The progressive changes in glomerular filtration rate which are associated with the evolution of nephropathy in type 1 diabetes patients are shown in Figure 10.1.

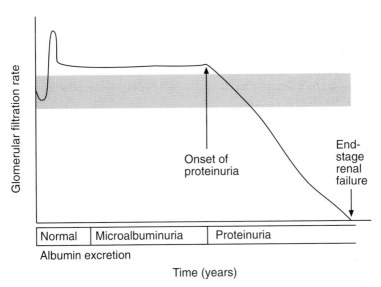

Figure 10.1 Natural history of diabetic nephropathy in type 1 diabetes. Shaded area equals normal range.

The earliest feature is thickening of the basement membrane which can be seen as early as two years after diagnosis. Expansion of mesangial tissues in the centre of the glomerulus leads to an increase in glomerular size, which then leads to an increase in overall kidney size. Changes in the size and structure of the filtration "pores" allow a gradual increase in urinary albumin excretion, initially termed microalbuminuria (see below). This progresses over 7–15 years to overt proteinuria which signals an inevitable deterioration of renal function to ESRF. During overt nephropathy, progressive scarring of glomeruli occurs as a result of ischaemia owing to mesangial expansion and occlusion of afferent arterioles.

As diabetic nephropathy progresses through these stages, a number of other characteristic clinical features develop, of which the most important is hypertension. These features are summarised in Box 10.1 and their clinical management is discussed below.

Type 2 diabetes

Much less is known of the natural history of nephropathy in type 2 diabetes, because it occurs in older patients, who often have co-existing hypertensive or renovascular disease or bladder outflow obstruction from prostatic disease, which complicates the natural history. For example, biopsy studies have shown that microalbuminuria is associated with typical diabetic glomerular disease in only one-third of cases. The rest have interstitial renovascular disease or tubular damage as a cause of microalbuminuria (see below). Similarly, in patients with end-stage disease requiring dialysis, a survey from King's College Hospital in London found that non-diabetic renal disease rather than diabetic nephropathy was responsible for over half of the cases of renal failure in type 2 diabetes.[7] In type 1 diabetes the figure was <10%.

The overall prevalence of microalbuminuria in type 2 diabetes is about 20% and prospective studies show that, as in type 1 diabetes, it predicts the development of overt proteinuria. However, it is also a strong independent predictor of cardiovascular death and, with the onset of overt proteinuria, this risk increases further. The natural history of renal disease is modified because many patients die from cardiovascular disease before ESRF develops.

Mortality risk and diabetic nephropathy

Persistent proteinuria is an ominous finding in both types of diabetes. Long-term studies suggest a median life expectancy of 10 years after the onset of proteinuria in type 1 diabetes, with two-thirds of deaths related to ESRF and one-third to cardiovascular

---

Box 10.1 Stages in the development of diabetic nephropathy

- *Hyperfiltration*
  - associated with increased glomerular size and kidney volume
  - increased glomerular filtration rate
  - may be reversible with good diabetic control

- *Microalbuminuria*
  - blood pressure increases relative to non-diabetic peers but usually remains below WHO criteria (<140/90)
  - early left ventricular hypertrophy
  - ACE inhibitors reduce microalbuminuria and may slow progression to established nephropathy

- *Established nephropathy*
  - progressive decline in renal function
  - worsening hypertension
  - Albustix-positive proteinuria occasionally with nephrotic syndrome
  - hyperlipidaemia
  - increased risk of ischaemic heart disease
  - high probability of proliferative diabetic retinopathy
  - early biochemical features of renal bone disease
  - aggressive antihypertensive therapy using ACE inhibitors in the treatment regimen slows the rate of decline of renal function

- *End-stage nephropathy*
  - renal failure needing dialysis or transplantation
  - widespread arterial disease
  - proliferative retinopathy and peripheral neuropathy common
  - 50% 3-year survival

---

disease. In type 2 diabetes, the risk of cardiovascular disease in those with overt proteinuria is so high that many die before they reach ESRF. The increased cardiovascular risk is partly explained by the effects of hypertension and hyperlipidaemia, which are commonly associated with proteinuria, but other factors, including smoking, obesity and defects in blood coagulation, are also likely to be implicated.

Screening and diagnosis of diabetic nephropathy

In all new patients with diabetes it is important to document previous renal disease and any family or personal history of hypertension or cardiovascular disease. Urinalysis should be performed for Albustix-positive proteinuria, and the serum urea and creatinine measured to establish baseline values. Supine and erect blood pressure readings should be recorded. Subsequently patients should be entered into a programme of annual checks to identify incipient nephropathy as soon as possible.

Microalbuminuria

Albumin can be detected in small amounts in the urine of healthy subjects. Microalbuminuria is a misnomer for urine albumin above the upper limit of normal but below the detection limit of Albustix test strips (Box 10.2). It is the earliest clinically detectable sign of diabetic nephropathy.

Box 10.2 Defining limits of microalbuminuria (albumin excretion rate per 24 h)

- Normal: 0–30 mg
- Microalbuminuria: 30–300 mg
- Overt proteinuria: >300 mg
- Nephrotic syndrome: >3000 mg

Within five years of diagnosis of type 1 diabetes, about 10% of patients have developed microalbuminuria and this approaches 50% after 30 years. Poor diabetic control, elevated blood pressure, and smoking are associated with a higher risk of microalbuminuria.[8] Microalbuminuria is important because it is a strong predictor of progression to established nephropathy, particularly when it develops within 10 years of diagnosis. Patients who develop microalbuminuria 20 or more years after diagnosis are less likely to progress.

The prevalence and natural history of microalbuminuria is less clearly defined in type 2 diabetes, but it is generally agreed that it confers a two- to three-fold increased risk of cardiovascular disease, independent of other conventional risk factors.

There is a considerable day-to-day variation in urine albumin excretion and, much as with blood pressure, several measurements are needed over a three to six month period to confirm persistent microalbuminuria. Current guidelines recommend an initial screening test that is best done by measuring the albumin concentration, corrected for creatinine, in an early morning urine sample (Table 10.1). Those with positive screening tests should be assessed with timed urine collections.

Table 10.1   Screening for microalbuminuria

Timing	Urine albumin creatinine ratio (mg/mmol)	
	Male	Female
Screening (Early morning)		
Normal	<2.5	<3.5
Borderline	2.5–7.0	3.5–10.0
Microalbuminuria	>7.5	>10.0
Confirmation		
Timed overnight:	20–200 μg/min	
or		
24-hour:	30–300 mg/24 h	

As urinary albumin excretion increases to >300 mg/day, it can be detected with reagent test strips such as Albustix. A reading of 1 + indicates an approximate 24-hour excretion of 500 mg of protein.

Clinical diagnosis of diabetic nephropathy

The diagnosis of diabetic nephropathy is usually straightforward in type 1 diabetes. The finding of proteinuria in a patient with a 10–20 year history of diabetes, associated with preproliferative or proliferative retinopathy, is typical. Renal biopsy adds nothing in such cases unless there is clinical or laboratory evidence of other conditions which may impair renal function.

The situation is often more complicated in type 2 diabetes because hypertension and vascular disease are more common. In men, bladder outflow obstruction is also an important differential diagnosis. As with type 1 diabetes, diabetic nephropathy is usually associated with moderate or severe retinopathy, although this is not always the case, particularly in patients from the Indian subcontinent. To avoid missing other potentially treatable renal diseases, it is worth doing some simple additional investigations in both types of diabetes as shown in Box 10.3.

Box 10.3 Investigations to exclude non-diabetic renal disease in a patient with diabetes and proteinuria

- Urine culture
  - exclude infection
- Urine microscopy
  - examine for red cell casts in glomerulonephritis
- Anti-DNA antibodies
- Complement levels
  - exclusion of autoimmune disease
- Rheumatoid factor
- Igs; protein electrophoretic strip
  - exclude multiple myeloma
- Renal ultrasound
  - assess renal anatomy and size
  - exclude obstructive renal disease

Renal biopsy

This should be reserved for patients in whom there is doubt about the diagnosis of diabetic nephropathy. Most commonly this situation arises in patients with renal disease but without diabetic retinopathy. It is also important to consider biopsy in patients with rapidly progressive renal disease. Red cell casts seen on microscopy may suggest active glomerulonephritis, although they have also been described in diabetic nephropathy.[9] Clinical features that would support renal biopsy in a patient with diabetes are summarised in Box 10.4.

Treatment of diabetic nephropathy

The emphasis in managing diabetic nephropathy is to protect renal function from the onset of diabetes and, when signs of

---

Box 10.4 Indications for renal biopsy in a patient with diabetes and proteinuria

- Short duration type 1 diabetes (<5 years)
- Clinical features of autoimmune disease which could involve the kidneys
- Mild or absent diabetic retinopathy
- Red cell casts in the urine
- Significant quantitative proteinuria (>2 g/24 h)

---

nephropathy are detected, to intervene in order to preserve it. As diabetic nephropathy progresses, new management issues arise and these will be discussed below.

Glycaemic control

Diabetic control is the major factor which determines progression from normal albumin excretion to microalbuminuria. Good diabetic control reduces the risk of microalbuminuria; in the Diabetes Control and Complications Trial,[10] the intensive cohort (mean HBA_{1c} 7.2%) had 39% less microalbuminuria than the conventional group (mean HBA_{1c} 9.2%.) How tight glycaemic control needs to be to reduce the risk of glomerular damage remains uncertain, but a recent study from the Mayo clinic[11] suggested a threshold effect, such that the risk of developing microalbuminuria increased significantly once mean HBA_{1c} went above 8.1% (HBA_1 10%) (Figure 10.2).

Other factors have been identified in prospective trials which increase the likelihood of developing microalbuminuria, including blood pressure, smoking and, possibly, serum LDL-cholesterol concentrations.

Whether improving diabetic control has a beneficial effect once patients have developed microalbuminuria is unclear. In the DCCT those with microalbuminuria at entry did not benefit from intensive glycaemic control, although numbers were too small to provide a definitive answer.[10] Most diabetologists would encourage patients to achieve as good glycaemic control as possible because, even if there is less to be gained from renal protection, the risk of other microvascular complications, such as retinopathy, can still be reduced.

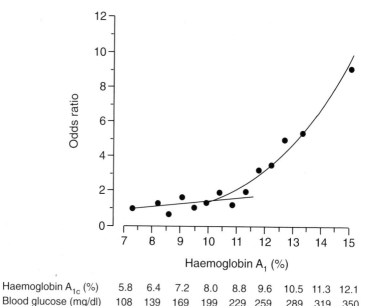

Haemoglobin A₁c (%)	5.8	6.4	7.2	8.0	8.8	9.6	10.5	11.3	12.1
Blood glucose (mg/dl)	108	139	169	199	229	259	289	319	350

Figure 10.2 Relation between mean haemoglobin A₁ values and the risk of microalbuminuria in patients with type 1 diabetes.

Microalbuminuria

Persistent microalbuminuria is associated with histological changes of early diabetic glomerulosclerosis in type 1 diabetes. It is also associated with raised blood pressure compared with patients with normal albumin excretion, although this does not usually reach WHO criteria for hypertension until the stage of overt proteinuria is reached.

ACE inhibitors have an established role in the treatment of microalbuminuria in type 1 diabetes. By reducing angiotensin II concentrations, they relax the efferent arteriole and hence lower intraglomerular pressure. In placebo-controlled trials, ACE inhibitors, at moderate to high dose, reduce progression of microalbuminuria in normotensive patients with type 1 diabetes (Table 10.2) and also in those who are hypertensive. Whether lower doses would provide the same benefit is unknown.

Normotensive patients should be started on an ACE inhibitor, once persistent microalbuminuria has been confirmed with several tests. Those with hypertension should also receive an ACE inhibitor

Table 10.2   Placebo-controlled trials assessing the effect of ACE inhibitors in progression of microalbuminuria to overt proteinuria in normotensive patients with type 1 diabetes

Study	n	Follow-up (years)	ACE	Dose	Progression to proteinuria			
					ACE (%)		Placebo (%)	
Marre et al.[12]	20	1	Enalapril	20 mg o.d.	0/10	(0)	3/10	(30)
Laffel & McGill[13]	143	2	Captopril	50 mg b.d.	4/67	(6)	13/70	(18.6)
MACG[14]	225	2	Captopril	25 mg b.d.	8/111	(7)	25/114	(21)

o.d. = once daily; b.d. = twice daily

as first line antihypertensive treatment; aim for a blood pressure of $\leqslant 130/85$. A few patients cannot tolerate ACE inhibitors mainly because of the side effect of cough. Other antihypertensives, including beta-blockers and non-dihydropyridine calcium antagonists (e.g. diltiazem), also reduce microalbuminuria, but long-term trials using these agents are more limited. ACE inhibitors are the only class of drug licensed for the treatment of microalbuminuria.

Persistent microalbuminuria in type 2 diabetes is a strong predictor of cardiovascular disease and, if it is present, patients should be screened for vascular risk factors and signs of established vascular disease and hypertension. Careful control of blood pressure is essential. Antihypertensive therapy must be tailored individually, but ACE inhibition is usually appropriate, although patients with concomitant disease may derive more benefit from a calcium channel blocker or cardioselective beta-blocker. Studies of ACE inhibition in microalbuminuric patients suggest a similar benefit on reducing urinary albumin excretion (Table 10.3).

In addition to assessing glycaemic control, investigations should include fasting total, HDL- and LDL-cholesterol, and triglycerides, and a resting ECG to look for evidence of ischaemia or ventricular hypertrophy. Treatment of cardiovascular risk factors is discussed in Chapter 7.

Overt diabetic nephropathy

Overt diabetic nephropathy is characterised by Albustix-positive proteinuria, hypertension, and a declining glomerular filtration rate. Progression to ESRF is inevitable, although the rate of deterioration

Table 10.3   Effect of ACE inhibitors in progress of microalbuminuria to overt proteinuria in patients with type 2 diabetes

Study	n	Follow-up (years)	ACE	Dose	Progression to proteinuria	
					ACE (%)	Placebo (%)
Ravid et al.[15]	94	5	Enalapril	10 mg o.d.	6/49 (12)	19/45 (42)
Sano et al.[16]	56	4	Enalapril	5 mg o.d.	0/28 (0)	8/28 (28)

o.d. = once daily

varies markedly between patients. The median time from onset of proteinuria to ESRF was about seven years in patients diagnosed with type 1 diabetes in the 1950s and 1960s. More recent evidence suggests that, with optimal management, this may be increased to 13–14 years.

Control of blood pressure undoubtedly offers the best chance of delaying ESRF. Studies in the 1980s showed that effective antihypertensive therapy with beta-blockers, diuretics, and vasodilators in established nephropathy slowed the rate of deterioration of renal function.[17] More recently, in a prospective trial involving over 400 patients with established nephropathy, ACE inhibition with captopril halved the progression to dialysis and transplantation, and reduced mortality by a similar percentage compared with placebo (Figure 10.3).[18] Blood pressure targets were set at ≤140/90, and other antihypertensive agents were used as clinically indicated.

A "no added salt" diet is advisable in patients on ACE inhibitors to maximise the hypotensive effects; as serum creatinine increases, adding a loop diuretic, such as frusemide, is often effective in maintaining control of blood pressure. Other antihypertensive combinations using beta-blockers, calcium channel blockers, or alpha-blockers, should be selected according to each patient's clinical profile. The target blood pressure should be ≤140/90, and combination therapy with three or more drugs is usually necessary.

Short-acting dihydropyridine calcium antagonists, such as nifedipine, may worsen proteinuria, and recent studies have suggested that they may have an adverse effect on cardiovascular mortality compared with ACE inhibition.[19,20] Non-dihydropyridine calcium antagonists, such as diltiazem or verapamil, are suitable alternatives. There is limited experience with angiotensin II

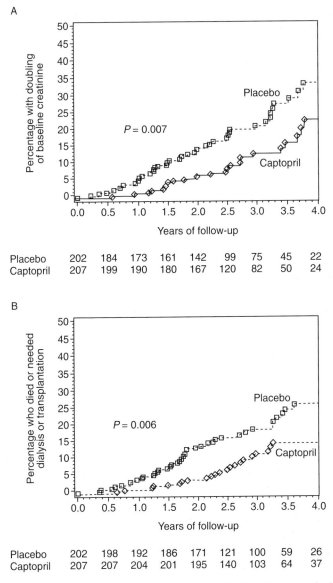

Figure 10.3 Cumulative incidence of events in patients with diabetic nephropathy in the captopril and placebo groups. Panel A shows the cumulative percentage of patients with the primary end-point; a doubling of the baseline serum creatinine concentration to at least 2.0 mg/dl. Panel B shows the cumulative percentage of patients who died or required dialysis or renal transplantation. The numbers at the bottom of each panel are the numbers of patients in each group at risk for the event at baseline and after each six-month period.

antagonists, although on theoretical grounds they may offer advantages over ACE inhibitors.

As diabetic nephropathy progresses fluid retention becomes a common problem that can worsen hypertension. Loop diuretics are helpful but large doses may be needed. It is sometimes necessary to add thiazide-type agents, such as metolazone.

Patients with established nephropathy need review every two to three months for monitoring of renal function, blood pressure, and fluid balance. Hypertension is often difficult to treat in progressive nephropathy. It is usual for combinations of three or four different antihypertensive drugs plus a diuretic to be used and, despite this, blood pressure targets of <140/90 may not be achievable. Compliance with such multiple tablet regimens can be a problem, and it is important to explain the potential benefits of treatment. Postural hypotension from autonomic neuropathy can make treatment of hypertension even more difficult. A patient may have significant hypertension when lying down, but may experience a precipitous fall in blood pressure on standing. Volume depletion from overdiuresis may compound the problem. For these reasons it is important to check lying *and* standing blood pressure at each review, and adjust antihypertensive and diuretic treatment accordingly.

With progression of nephropathy and a rising serum creatinine, the renal clearance of insulin declines and patients become more insulin-sensitive. Insulin doses usually need to be progressively reduced, according to results of HBA_{1c} and capillary blood glucose testing, sometimes by as much as 30–50% overall, to avoid hypoglycaemia (see Chapter 4).

Oral hypoglycaemic medication also needs to be reviewed as nephropathy progresses. Since most sulphonylureas (or their metabolites) are renally excreted, they accumulate as renal function declines, increasing the risk of hypoglycaemia (see Chapter 4). Second generation sulphonylureas, such as gliclazide, which are hepatically-metabolised, are safer, and can be continued providing glycaemic control is satisfactory. Metformin is renally excreted and, when serum creatinine concentrations are >150 μmol/litre, it should be stopped, because of the increased risk of lactic acidosis. This often precipitates a switch to insulin, particularly in patients who are already taking metformin in combination with high doses of a sulphonylurea. Most patients should be transferred to insulin as serum creatinine rises >200 μmol/litre, because it provides greater flexibility for diabetic control during dialysis.

Established nephropathy and renal osteodystrophy

As serum creatinine ⩾150 μmol/litre, hyperphosphataemia and hypocalcaemia develop as a result of reduced renal phosphate clearance. Hypocalcaemia stimulates parathyroid hormone secretion, with the progressive development of hyperparathyroid bone disease in a proportion of diabetic patients with progressive renal failure.

Serum calcium, phosphate, alkaline phosphate, and albumin should be measured every six months. Treatment with an oral phosphate binding agent, such as calcium carbonate (Titralac), to control hyperphosphataemia should be started when phosphate increases above the normal range. Rising bone alkaline phosphatase concentrations are a useful sign of developing hyperparathyroid bone disease and should prompt the measurement of serum parathyroid hormone (PTH). If PTH concentrations are raised, treatment with 0.25–0.5 μg of 1-alpha hydroxyvitamin D should be started with regular monitoring of serum calcium concentrations.

Established nephropathy and cardiovascular risk

Patients with proteinuria are at high risk of cardiovascular disease and attention must be paid to treatable risk factors. Control of diabetes and hypertension has already been discussed, and smoking should be strongly discouraged in all patients. Lipid profiles are often abnormal in diabetic nephropathy. Typically total and LDL-cholesterol and triglycerides are raised and HDL-cholesterol is reduced, and this may contribute to the high prevalence of macrovascular disease in diabetic nephropathy. Statins are the treatment of choice since they are metabolised by the liver and do not accumulate in renal failure. They also have a proven benefit in cardiovascular protection and it is reasonable to start treatment if the total or LDL-cholesterol remains >5.5 mmol/litre or 4.1 mmol/litre respectively. Fibrates should not be used in renal impairment because they can accumulate in renal failure and increase the risk of myositis.

Preparation for renal replacement therapy

This takes time and patients should be referred to renal services sufficiently early in their clinical course to allow the necessary preparations to be completed. A useful rule of thumb is to refer once the serum creatinine has increased to >200 μmol/litre, or when renal replacement is anticipated within the next year. The rate of change of serum creatinine is very variable between patients and an estimate of the likely time to dialysis can be obtained from the slope of the inverse creatinine plot; this is reliable once the serum creatinine is >150 μmol/litre (Figure 10.4).

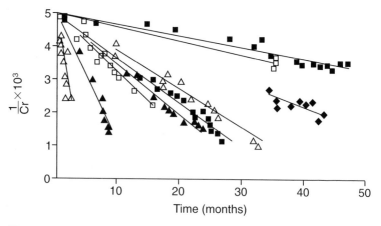

Figure 10.4 Progression of renal failure in nine diabetic patients—inverse of serum creatinine (μmol/litre) plotted against time.

When creatinine rises to >200 μmol/litre, some patients develop electrolyte abnormalities, particularly hyperkalaemia, that can be exacerbated by ACE inhibition. A low potassium diet can be helpful to control hyperkalaemia and allow the continuation of the ACE inhibitor. Dietary protein restriction has been advocated as a way of preserving renal function, although there is no conclusive evidence to support this in man. Moderate protein restriction can help to limit uraemic symptoms as renal failure progresses.

There are several issues which should be resolved for the preparation for future renal replacement therapy (Box 10.5). Ideally clinical management of these complicated patients should be jointly supervised by a diabetologist, renal physician, diabetes and renal nurse specialists, and a dietitian, so that renal management can be planned whilst other complications, including retinopathy, neuropathy, and macrovascular disease, are not forgotten.

Box 10.5 Reasons for early referral to a renal physician

- Psychological adjustment of the patient to impending dialysis
- Advice about low potassium and low protein diets
- Decision about which type of dialysis is most appropriate
- Hepatitis B immunisation
- Tissue typing/assessment for renal transplantation
- Vascular access for haemodialysis
- Assessment for erythropoietin therapy.

There has been a progressive increase in the numbers of patients with diabetes who are accepted onto renal replacement programmes, and they now constitute about one-third of the workload of most renal units. Most of this new demand is due to the inclusion of older patients with type 2 diabetes. The outlook for such patients has improved markedly in the last 20 years but, in general, the prognosis of patients with diabetes remains less optimistic than in non-diabetics, because of severe coexistent medical problems. There are three ways of treating ESRF— peritoneal dialysis, haemodialysis and transplantation.

Continuous ambulatory peritoneal dialysis (CAPD)

This offers particular advantages for the diabetic patient since it does not produce marked fluctuations of blood pressure and extracellular volume. Fluid balance is maintained with a combination of isotonic (weak) and hypertonic (strong) dialysate solutions which are poured into the abdominal cavity through a catheter in the anterior abdominal wall. Three or four bag changes are required every day, with each bag taking about 20 minutes to empty. Diabetic control can be maintained by adding insulin to the dialysate fluid. Because the dialysate contains glucose as an osmotic agent, the total daily dose of insulin usually needs to be doubled, with higher doses being used for the hypertonic bags than the isotonic bags. Peritonitis is the major complication of CAPD and is discussed in Chapter 11. CAPD is an effective long-term treatment for ESRF in diabetes, particularly in patients who are unsuitable for renal transplantation. Blind patients and the elderly can usually manage CAPD, provided they do not have other severe complications.

Haemodialysis

Haemodialysis requires several months' preparation in order to obtain vascular access through fashioning of an arteriovenous fistula. Patency rates of fistulae are lower and they take longer to mature than in non-diabetics. Patients usually need three dialysis sessions every week, each lasting two to three hours. Insulin requirements usually increase when haemodialysis is started and it can be difficult to maintain stable diabetic control. Fluctuations in blood pressure and extracellular fluid volume are also a problem in diabetic patients on haemodialysis, particularly if there is significant autonomic neuropathy which exacerbates postural hypotension. Long-term survival with haemodialysis is approximately 80% at one year and 40% at five years.[21]

Transplantation

With careful patient selection, renal transplantation is the treatment of choice. Survival for live donor transplants is on a par with non-diabetics and a successful transplant offers the best opportunity for effective rehabilitation. Contraindications include serious cardio- or cerebrovascular disease, and significant ongoing infection; most centres do not transplant patients over 65 years. Preparation for transplantation is similar to that for non-diabetics and includes blood grouping, tissue typing, hepatitis B immunisation, and careful assessment for a possible live related donor. Patients also need to be carefully screened for other diabetic micro- and macrovascular complications.

Nephrotic syndrome

The nephrotic syndrome is an uncommon but serious manifestation of diabetic nephropathy, usually associated with a poor prognosis due to rapid progression to end-stage renal failure. It may also suggest an alternative cause of renal disease such as minimal change or IgA nephropathy, and renal biopsy may be necessary to clarify this difficult diagnostic problem. Nephrotic range proteinuria presents with the onset of marked oedema secondary to hypoalbuminaemia and control of fluid balance presents particular problems in management, as is illustrated in the following case.

Case Study 30

A 27-year-old woman developed type 1 diabetes at the age of 9 years. Her diabetic control had been poor since diagnosis, with HBA_1 results ranging between 11–17%. She developed proliferative retinopathy 10 years after diagnosis treated with photocoagulation. Two years later, persistent proteinuria was noted. Her blood pressure was 130/94 mmHg and she was treated with enalapril 20 mg/day. She remained well for three years, but presented acutely with a three-week history of progressive ankle swelling and periorbital oedema. Investigations revealed proteinuria of 3.4 g/24 h with a serum albumin of 24 g/dl. Her serum creatinine was normal and her blood pressure 130/94 mmHg. She was treated with frusemide 250 mg/day, spironolactone 100 mg twice daily, and metolazone 5 mg once or twice weekly according to weight. The enalapril was increased to 20 mg twice daily.

Over the next two years her proteinuria increased to >8 g/24 h, and she required continued high-dose oral diuretics to control fluid retention. Stable fluid balance was difficult to maintain and she was advised to adjust the frequency of metolazone tablets according to how her weight compared with an estimated "dry weight". Even so, she required three further admissions, two of which were the result of fluid retention and one of overdiuresis with postural hypotension. She continued to take maximum doses of enalapril but, owing to the fluctuations in fluid balance, it was difficult to achieve stable blood pressure control. Her serum cholesterol increased to 9.4 mmol/litre; for which she was treated with simvastatin.

Her serum creatinine gradually increased and she was referred to the local renal unit when it exceeded 200 μmol/litre. Investigations did not suggest an alternative cause of the nephrotic syndrome, and renal biopsy was not performed because of the presence of associated microvascular complications. Anticipating the need for renal replacement therapy within the next 12 months, she was referred for assessment for transplantation and fashioning of a fistula for future haemodialysis.

Treatment of the nephrotic syndrome revolves around control of fluid balance and blood pressure. Loop diuretics are usually required, and high doses, ranging from 120 to 1000 mg/day of frusemide or its equivalent, are usually required with the addition of agents such as metolazone. Overdiuresis is an ever-present risk, and is usually associated with a reversible deterioration of renal function.

Control of hypertension is important in preserving renal function and, if tolerated, an ACE inhibitor should be included in the antihypertensive regimen. Blood pressure should always be measured with the patient supine and erect, since symptomatic postural hypotension can impose limitations on supine blood pressure control. Lipid-lowering therapy with a statin is usually necessary.

Unlike "garden-type" diabetic nephropathy, in which there are arguments to support dietary protein restriction on the grounds that it may preserve renal function, in the nephrotic syndrome a high protein diet (>100 g/day) is recommended in an attempt to maintain serum protein levels and minimise oedema.

Pregnancy and diabetic renal disease

With modern obstetric care and optimal diabetic control before and during pregnancy, perinatal outcomes of women who do not have advanced diabetic complications are similar to those in non-diabetic women. The outlook for women with overt nephropathy who become pregnant is less optimistic. A 10-year survey of pregnancies of women with nephropathy in Germany highlights many of the potential problems. From the first to the third trimester the percentage of women with nephrotic range proteinuria (>3 g/day) increased from 14 to 53%, and those treated with antihypertensive medication increased from 50 to 97%. One third of babies were born before 34 weeks, and 25% had respiratory distress syndrome.[22] The case report below illustrates some of the potential management problems.

Case Study 31

A 32-year-old woman with a 22-year history of type 1 diabetes, complicated by proliferative retinopathy, peripheral neuropathy and nephropathy, presented for antenatal care. She had developed proteinuria 12 years after diagnosis and her serum creatinine had remained normal for a further three years. She had a creatinine clearance of 66 ml/min (normal >100 ml/min) five years previously and had been treated with an ACE inhibitor and diuretics. Diabetic control had been poor with HBA_{1c} results ranging between 9 and 12%, and she had several previous admissions with ketoacidosis. She was para 7, gravida 2. Her youngest child had been born three years previously at 27 weeks gestation because of hypertension and oedema. Renal function at that time showed a creatinine clearance of 22 ml/min and a 24-hour protein excretion of 2.8 g. She had been advised of the risks of future pregnancies at that stage.

On this occasion she was 13 weeks pregnant at presentation. Her creatinine was 179 µmol/litre, and her creatinine clearance 36 ml/min. The ACE inhibitor was stopped and methyldopa commenced for control of hypertension, together with aspirin for prophylaxis against pre-eclampsia. She managed to improve her diabetic control, achieving an HBA_{1c} of 7% in the second trimester. Her 24-hour urine excretion ranged between 1.6 and 3 g/day and she continued to take loop diuretics to control her oedema. She required admission at 24 weeks for uncontrolled hypertension which responded to rest and increased doses of methyldopa. At 29 weeks she had spontaneous rupture of membranes and was delivered of a baby weighing 1.06 kg. The baby spent three months on neonatal intensive care.

Post-delivery ACE inhibition was reintroduced, together with her maintenance loop diuretic. She agreed to laparoscopic sterilisation. Her serum creatinine remained stable at 198 µmol/litre and her creatinine clearance had fallen to 15 ml/min; she was referred for a preliminary appointment to the renal services.

Pregnancy does not worsen renal function in the long-term, but women with nephropathy have a greatly increased risk of increased proteinuria, oedema, and hypertension during the pregnancy which usually has to be controlled with diuretics and antihypertensive drugs, such as methyldopa or nifedipine. Patients on ACE inhibition before conception should stop this treatment once pregnancy is confirmed. ACE inhibitors have no proven teratogenic effects but they can affect fetal renal function if they are continued into the third trimester. They should be reintroduced after delivery.

The creatinine level and blood pressure at conception is a useful guide to the potential outcome of the pregnancy. Serum creatinine <175 µmol/litre and diastolic blood pressure <90 mmHg are usually associated with a successful pregnancy, whereas if creatinine levels are >250 µmol/litre, fewer than half of the pregnancies have a successful outcome.

The long-term maternal prognosis depends on the severity of the renal disease. Of the 29 mothers described by Kimmerle and colleagues, eight had developed ESRF needing dialysis during an average of three years follow-up, of whom four had died.[22] An important part of postnatal care in women with nephropathy is to discuss the risks of future pregnancies and advise on appropriate contraceptive measures.

Renovascular disease

Renal artery stenosis (RAS) is an important macrovascular complication which is usually associated with hypertension and a progressive deterioration of renal function. It is more common in diabetes, particularly those with type 2; in a study of over 5000 post mortems, 8.3% of patients with diabetes had RAS compared with an overall prevalence of 4.3%.[23] In many cases the diagnosis had not been considered during life. RAS is more likely to be found in patients with clinical evidence of vascular disease elsewhere, particularly in the lower limbs; those with vascular disease affecting five or more peripheral vessels have a six- to seven-fold increased chance of having RAS compared with those having one- or two-vessel disease.

The possibility of RAS is an important clinical consideration in choosing appropriate antihypertensive agents. In the presence of bilateral RAS, ACE inhibitors may precipitate acute renal failure. Care should be taken in starting these drugs in patients with widespread vascular disease, and serum creatinine should always be checked before and 7–14 days after starting therapy in such patients.

Clinically significant RAS should be suspected in patients with hypertension and deteriorating renal function. Initial investigations should include a renal ultrasound which may show a small kidney in unilateral disease; colour-flow Doppler studies can provide a non-invasive assessment of renal artery flow. Arteriography remains the "gold standard" investigation, and may be combined with percutaneous transluminal balloon angioplasty (PTCA) in cases where renal function is deteriorating. In these circumstances PTCA may stabilise renal function, but improvement occurs in only a small minority. Long-term follow-up of patients with diabetes undergoing PTCA remains limited but, in general, they do less well than non-diabetics. About 50% achieve stabilisation of renal function in the first year following PTCA compared with 75% of non-diabetics.

Hyporeninaemic hypoaldosteronism

In this condition the normal renin response to standing or salt restriction is impaired, causing hypoaldosteronism with resulting hyperkalaemia. The cause is poorly understood but damage to the juxtaglomerular apparatus or the macula densa cells has been suggested. It is relatively common in patients with diabetic nephropathy and is characterised by persistent hyperkalaemia with a hyperchloraemic metabolic acidosis. On occasion it can present as life-threatening hyperkalaemia as is shown in the following case.

Case Study 32

A 76-year-old man with a 12-year history of type 2 diabetes was admitted as an emergency, having suffered a sudden collapse. He had been given emergency resuscitation from a member of the public who had realised that he was pulseless. The paramedic team found that he was pulseless with no spontaneous respiration. His cardiographic trace showed ventricular fibrillation and, after intubation, he was successfully cardioverted. He was transferred urgently to the local A&E department. On arrival he was semiconscious but was maintaining an adequate cardiac output; he showed no focal neurological signs. Urgent biochemistry revealed a serum potassium of 8.4 mmol/litre, together with a raised serum urea and creatinine. The blood glucose was 17.4 mmol/litre. Cardiac enzymes were not raised, and the ECG showed typical features of hyperkalaemia only. He had recently been prescribed a non-steroidal anti-inflammatory drug by his general practitioner.

He was treated with an intravenous bolus of 10 ml 10% calcium gluconate followed by an infusion of 100 ml 20% glucose and 15 units soluble insulin over one hour. His ECG improved and his serum potassium fell to 6.8 mmol/litre one hour later. The glucose/insulin treatment was repeated and his serum potassium subsequently fell to <6 mmol/litre. His ACE inhibitor and NSAID tablets were stopped. Over the next few days his serum potassium remained between 6 and 6.5 mmol/litre, and he had a low serum bicarbonate of 16 mmol/litre. A short synacthen test to exclude adrenal failure was normal. Measurement of serum renin and aldosterone revealed low concentrations of each, and a diagnosis of hyporeninaemic hypoaldosteronism was made. Hyperkalaemia was thought to have been exacerbated by the NSAID medication. He was started on fludrocortisone, 100 μg/day, which lowered his serum potassium into the normal range.

Hyporeninaemic hypoaldosteronism is the commonest cause of chronic hyperkalaemia[24] in diabetes, but it is important, as in the case described above, to exclude other causes, including overzealous potassium replacement, spironolactone treatment, haemolysis, and adrenal failure. Once the diagnosis is confirmed by measurement of serum renin and aldosterone, treatment with fludrocortisone should correct the hyperkalaemia.

References

1 Raine AEG. Evolution worldwide of the treatment of patients with advanced diabetic nephropathy by renal replacement therapy. In: Mogensen CE, ed. *The kidney and hypertension in diabetes mellitus.* Boston: Kluwer Academic Publishers, 1994:449–58.

2 Krowlewski M, Eggars P, Warram JH. Magnitude of end-stage renal disease in IDDM: a 35 year follow-up study. *Kidney Internat* 1996;**50**: 2041–6.

3 Ordonez JD, Hiatt RA. Comparison of Type-II and Type-I diabetics treated for end-stage-renal disease in a large prepaid health plan population. *Nephron* 1989;**51**:524–9.

4 Burden AC, McNally P, Feehally J *et al.* Increased incidence of end-stage-renal-failure secondary to diabetes mellitus in Asian ethnic groups in the United Kingdom. *Diabetic Med* 1992;**9**:641–5.

5 Cowie CC, Port FK, Wolfe RA *et al.* Disparities in incidence of diabetic end-stage renal disease according to race and type of diabetes. *New Engl J Med* 1989;**321**:1074–9.

6 Seaquist ER, Goetz FC, Rich S *et al.* Familial clustering of diabetic kidney disease: evidence of genetic susceptibility to diabetic nephropathy. *New Engl J Med* 1989;**320**:1161–5.

7 Grenfell A, Bewick M, Snowden S *et al.* Renal replacement therapy for diabetic patients: experience at King's College Hospital 1980–1989. *Q J Med* 1992;**85**:861–74.

8 Microalbuminuria Collaborative Study Group, United Kingdom. Risk factors for development of microalbuminuria in insulin-dependent diabetic patients: a cohort study. *Br Med J* 1993;**306**:1235–9.

9 O'Neill WM Jr, Wallin JD, Walker PD. Haematuria and red cell casts in typical diabetic nephropathy. *Am J Med* 1983;**74**:389–95.

10 Diabetes Control and Complications Trial Research Group. Effect of intensive therapy on the development and progression of diabetic nephropathy in the diabetes control and complications trial. *Kidney Internat* 1995;**47**:1703–20.

11 Krowlewski AS, Laffel LMB, Krowlewski M, Quinn M, Warram JH. Glycated haemoglobin and risk of microalbuminuria in patients with insulin-dependent diabetes mellitus. *New Engl J Med* 1995;**332**: 1251–5.

12 Marre M, Chatellier G, Leblanc H *et al.* Prevention of diabetic nephropathy with enalapril in normotensive diabetics with micro-albuminuria. *Br Med J* 1988;**297**:1092–5.

13 Laffel MB, McGill JB for the North American Microalbuminuria Study Group. The beneficial effect of angiotensin-converting enzyme inhibition with captopril on diabetic nephropathy in normotensive IDDM patients with microalbuminuria. *Am J Med* 1995;**99**:497–504.

14 Microalbuminuria Captopril Study Group. Captopril reduces the risk of nephropathy in IDDM patients with microalbuminuria. *Diabetologia* 1996;**39**:587–93.

15 Ravid M, Savin H, Jutrin I *et al.* Long-term stabilizing effect of angiotensin-converting enzyme inhibition on plasma creatinine and on proteinuria in normotensive Type II diabetic patients. *Ann Intern Med* 1993;**118**:577–81.

16 Sano T, Hotta N, Kawamura T, Matsumae H *et al.* Effects of long-term enalapril treatment on persistent microalbuminuria in normotensive Type-2 diabetic patients: results of a 4-year, prospective randomised study. *Diabetic Med* 1996;**13**:120–4.

17 Parving HH, Andersen AR, Smidt UM *et al.* Effect of antihypertensive treatment on kidney function in diabetic nephropathy *Br Med J* 1987; **294**:1443–7.

18 Lewis EJ, Hunsickler LG, Bain RP, Rohde RD. The effect of angiotensin converting enzyme inhibition on diabetic nephropathy. *New Engl J Med* 1993;**329**:1456–62.

19 Estacio RO, Jeffers BW, Hiatt WR *et al.* The effect of nisoldipine as compared with enalapril on cardiovascular outcomes in patients with non-insulin-dependent diabetes and hypertension. *New Engl J Med* 1998;**338**:645–52.

20 Tatti P, Pahor M, Byington RP *et al.* Outcome results of the fosinopril versus amlodipine cardiovascular events randomised trial (FACET) in patients with hypertension and NIDDM. *Diabetes Care* 1998;**21**: 597–603.

21 Koch M, Thomas B, Tschope W *et al.* Survival and predictors of death in dialysed diabetics. *Diabetologia* 1993;**36**:1113–17.

22 Kimmerle R, Zab R-P, Cupisti S *et al.* Pregnancies in women with diabetic nephropathy: long-term outcome for mother and child. *Diabetologia* 1995;**38**:227–35.

23 Sawicki PT, Kaiser S, Heinemann L, Frenzel H, Berger M. Prevalence of renal artery stenosis in diabetes mellitus—an autopsy study. *J Intern Med* 1991;**229**:489–92.

24 Tan SY, Burton M. Hyporeninaemic hypoaldosteronism. An overlooked cause of hyperkalaemia. *Arch Intern Med* 1981;**141**:30–3.

11 Diabetes and infections

Patients with poorly controlled diabetes are more susceptible to both common and exotic bacterial and fungal infections.[1] There are several reasons for this. Firstly hyperglycaemia impairs neutrophil functions including chemotaxis, phagocytosis, and bactericidal activity, which may reduce host defences against infection. Skin carriage with *Staphylococcus aureus* is also more common in patients with type 1 diabetes, and this increases the likelihood of soft tissue infection when there is trauma to the skin. A typical site for such infection is the neuropathic foot in which microvascular disease and poor capillary perfusion of the skin may further reduce the normal responses to infection. In addition to these clinical problems, there are some potentially life-threatening infections that occur almost exclusively in patients with diabetes.[2]

Acute infection is associated with stress hormone responses causing hyperglycaemia and occasionally ketoacidosis. There is no hard evidence that tight glycaemic control influences prognosis in severe infections but, most clinicians would try to achieve this. This may involve switching patients with type 2 diabetes to insulin as a temporary measure, and it is sometimes necessary to use an intravenous sliding scale insulin regimen (Chapter 2).

This chapter considers the diagnosis and management of potentially serious infections which occur more commonly in patients with diabetes. Infection in the diabetic foot is described in Chapter 8.

Urinary tract

Lower urinary tract infection

Cystitis is more common in women with diabetes and, in addition to causing local symptoms, may upset diabetic control. Gram negative or anaerobic organisms are the usual pathogens, and risk of infection is increased with age, disease duration and impaired bladder emptying from autonomic neuropathy. Early treatment with appropriate antibiotics is necessary to reduce the risk of ascending infection. Urine should be recultured after treatment to check that the infection has been eradicated. Recurrence is common and repeated infections should prompt investigation of the renal tract with ultrasound to exclude anatomical problems, papillary necrosis, renal stone disease, and incomplete bladder emptying. Occasionally long-term low-dose antibiotics are necessary to prevent repeated episodes of cystitis.

Pyelonephritis

Pyelonephritis usually presents with typical symptoms of loin pain, fever, and rigors, often associated with marked metabolic disturbance. Gram negative rods are by far the commonest organisms, and the diagnosis is confirmed by culture of urine and blood. Intravenous antibiotics are given, with third-generation cephalosporins as first-line agents. Rarely pyelonephritis may cause parenchymal abscess formation as is shown in the following case.

Case Study 33

A 51-year-old woman with long-standing type 1 diabetes was admitted with a short history of vomiting, right-sided loin pain, and fever with rigors. Her diabetic control had been poor as a result of the illness with marked hyperglycaemia. Examination confirmed right loin tenderness and a fever. A clinical diagnosis of right-sided pyelonephritis was made and she was started on intravenous antibiotics with an insulin sliding scale. Subsequently *Klebsiella* sp. was grown from both blood and urine cultures. Her general condition and fever initially improved, but she developed recurrent loin pain and a fluctuating temperature despite continued antibiotics. Ultrasound revealed the right kidney to be enlarged with several hypoechoic areas within the renal cortex. There was no evidence of obstruction. CT scanning suggested multifocal abscesses. Treatment with high-dose intravenous antibiotics was continued and the patient gradually improved. Repeat CT scanning showed resolution of the abscesses. After six weeks the antibiotics were stopped and repeat cultures were negative. There have been no subsequent recurrences.

219

In most cases of renal abscess formation, a prolonged course of antibiotics will lead to resolution, but percutaneous or open drainage should be considered after a few days, if there is no clinical improvement with antibiotics.

Cortical abscesses, otherwise known as renal carbuncles, usually occur as a result of haematogenous spread of *Staphylococcus aureus* infection from a distant site. Presentation is similar to cortico-medullary abscesses and treatment is with a prolonged course of appropriate high dose intravenous antibiotics. Surgical drainage is occasionally required.

Perinephric abscess occurs when infection spreads from par-enchymal renal abscesses beyond the renal capsule and is more common with diabetes. CT scanning is the best investigation and, if the diagnosis is confirmed, percutaneous drainage is usually necessary, in combination with a prolonged course of antibiotics.

Papillary necrosis

This occurs when the renal papillae lose their blood supply and slough into the pelvicalyceal system. It is a rare complication of pyelonephritis and usually presents with clinical features of persistent or recurrent pyelonephritis that proves difficult to eradicate, as illustrated in the following case.

Case Study 34

A 75-year-old previously fit woman with insulin-treated type 2 diabetes was admitted with a fever, left-sided loin pain, and hypotension. She had a five-day history of frequency and dysuria. She was confused and disorientated. Examination revealed her to be very unwell with a pulse of 120 bpm, atrial fibrillation, a systolic blood pressure of 80 mmHg, and marked left loin tenderness. She had a raised white cell count with a neutrophilia and impaired renal function (urea of 26 mmol/litre, creatinine 220 μmol/litre).

She was treated with intravenous fluids and broad spectrum antibiotics. *Escherichia coli* was subsequently grown in all blood culture bottles and from her urine. Her temperature settled and renal function gradually improved with rehydration, but did not return to normal.

Five days later she deteriorated with recurrent loin pain, fever, and oliguria. An urgent renal ultrasound showed obstruction of the left kidney at the pelvicalyceal junction, and a percutaneous nephrostomy was inserted with drainage of purulent urine. Her serum creatinine rose to 630 μmol/litre over the next few days as a result of infection and probable acute tubular necrosis. She developed terminal bronchopneumonia and died two days later. A post-mortem confirmed severe ischaemic change in the kidneys with papillary infarction and necrosis.

About 50% of cases of papillary necrosis occur in patients with diabetes, with the greatest risk seen in middle-aged or elderly women. It may also complicate sickle cell disease and analgesic abuse. It should be suspected when loin pain and fever persist despite appropriate antibiotics. Microscopic haematuria and pyuria are common, and the diagnosis can be confirmed with renal ultrasound or CT scanning, although retrograde pyelography is the investigation of choice. Treatment usually involves prolonged antibiotics and measures to treat renal impairment, if this develops. Occasionally, as in the above case, renal obstruction occurs which needs percutaneous drainage to preserve renal function.

Continuous ambulatory peritoneal dialysis (CAPD)

End-stage diabetic nephropathy is commonly treated with CAPD. Infective peritonitis is a well-recognised complication of CAPD as a result of infection of the indwelling catheter, or contamination of the dialysate fluid from poor technique. A typical case is described.

Case Study 35

A 45-year-old man with long-standing type 1 diabetes was admitted for treatment of an ischaemic foot ulcer. He had developed end-stage renal failure five years previously and had had two renal transplants, both of which had failed due to rejection. He had resumed CAPD six months before. During his admission he complained of feeling non-specifically unwell, with mild abdominal discomfort and a temperature of 37.5–38°C. There was no sign of acute infection around his catheter site but the dialysate fluid was noted to be cloudy and, on microscopy, found to contain over 1000 cells/mm^3. Culture grew a coagulase-negative staphylococcus. He was treated with intravenous and subsequently oral antibiotics for 10 days and rapidly improved.

Gram positive organisms including streptococci and staphylococci are responsible for about 60% of cases of peritonitis, with gram negative organisms accounting for most other cases. Occasionally fungal infection with *Candida* spp. are isolated. As in the above case, symptoms are usually mild. It is important to examine the catheter insertion site, since this may be the source of infection, and to check the patient's bag changing technique. Cloudiness of the dialysate fluid is usual and samples should be sent for culture to confirm the diagnosis. In many cases antibiotic treatment can be given on an outpatient basis, and some centres recommend adding antibiotics to the dialysate bag.

Penile implants

Rigid or inflatable penile implants are associated with a 2–3% rate of infection in most series, with *Staphylococcus epidermidis* or coliforms the most likely organisms. Symptoms range from mild tenderness to severe induration, with fistula formation and erosion of the implant through the skin of the penis. Treatment involves surgical removal of the device with appropriate broad spectrum antibiotics. Rarely, intracavernosal injection therapy can also cause severe staphylococcal infection, particularly if aseptic technique is poor.[3]

Soft tissue and bone infection

Malignant otitis externa

The following case illustrates a case of malignant otitis externa.

Case Study 36

A 52-year-old man with type 2 diabetes presented to the medical on-call team with severe left-sided facial pain. He had attended his local ENT department for treatment of a left middle ear infection for three weeks and had developed a thick white fluid discharge three days before admission. Examination revealed treated proliferative retinopathy and peripheral neuropathy. Two toes on his left foot had been amputated three years previously. There were no neurological findings.

Swabs of the external auditory canal grew *Pseudomonas aeruginosa*. A cranial CT scan, to exclude a cerebral abscess, was normal, and a diagnosis of otitis externa was made. He was treated with antibiotic drops and analgesia, and discharged with further ENT outpatient review. Two weeks later his symptoms persisted, and he was admitted for left mastoid exploration under anaesthetic. A mass of polypoid granulations found arising from the middle ear cleft were removed. Material obtained at surgery grew *Pseudomonas aeruginosa* but, since his pain was improved postoperatively, antibiotics were not started. Two weeks later his severe constant facial pain recurred and he needed urgent re-admission. On this occasion an isotope bone scan was performed, which showed extensive uptake in the left temporal bone. A CT scan showed extensive inflammatory disease in the mastoid with erosion of the adjacent temporomandibular joint. He was started on high-dose ciprofloxacin but, over the following two weeks, his condition deteriorated. He developed a left-sided facial nerve palsy and one week later complained of difficulty swallowing; he was noted to have a hoarse voice. A left palatal paralysis was noted. Despite high-dose antibiotics, he developed progressive dysphagia and marked weight loss, and he required enteral feeding. He died from a complicating bronchopneumonia.

Malignant otitis externa is a chronic osteomyelitis of the base of the skull that particularly affects elderly patients with diabetes.[4] Almost all cases are associated with *Pseudomonas aeruginosa* infection that starts in the external auditory canal and spreads between the cartilaginous and osseous parts of the canal to involve the temporal bone and eventually the base of the skull. The above case is typical in that the patient experiences unrelenting severe pain in the auditory canal with associated temporal headache. Facial nerve involvement is common, affecting up to 50% of cases; other cranial nerves may also be involved as the osteomyelitis extends into the base of the skull.

The diagnosis should be suspected in any elderly patient with type 2 diabetes who presents with a chronic ear discharge that grows *Pseudomonas aeruginosa* on culture. Inflammatory markers, including ESR (erythrocyte sedimentation rate) and CRP (C-reactive protein), are usually increased. Technetium bone scanning is sensitive but lacks specificity, and either CT or MR scanning is the radiological investigation of choice.

Early reports suggested a near 100% mortality but, more recently, with earlier diagnosis and the introduction of improved anti-pseudomonal antibiotics, this has fallen to 10–20%. High-dose intravenous antipseudomonal antibiotics are recommended in most cases, particularly with cranial nerve involvement but, with early diagnosis and a compliant patient, a prolonged course of oral ciprofloxacin has been shown to be effective.[5] Antibiotic treatment should continue for four to eight weeks. Local debridement of granulation tissue in the external auditory canal may be required. Monitoring should include clinical response, serial imaging, and changes in inflammatory markers. Late diagnosis, short or inappropriate courses of antibiotics, and progressive cranial nerve involvement are associated with a poor prognosis.

Spinal abscess

Vertebral osteomyelitis is a rare cause of back pain that occurs more commonly in patients with diabetes than in the general population. A recently published survey from Denmark suggested a significant increase in frequency during the 1980s.[6] It usually affects patients >50 years of age and between 10 and 20% will have diabetes.

Staphylococcus aureus is the most common infecting organism and there are often few clinical clues as to the source of the infection.[7] The following case report illustrates some of the clinical features and management of this difficult condition.

Case Study 37

A 50-year-old man with long-standing type 1 diabetes complicated by retinopathy, peripheral neuropathy, and vascular disease was admitted with a one-week history of increasingly severe pain in the region of his right scapula, associated with malaise and fever. He had been a recent inpatient for treatment of a neuroischaemic ulcer with osteomyelitis, and his left hallux had been amputated. On readmission he was febrile, with a necrotic area around the amputation site. There was a full range of shoulder movements, but he had some localised tenderness of the cervical spine. Investigations revealed raised inflammatory markers and white count with a neutrophilia. Chest and shoulder radiographs were normal. *Staphylococcus aureus* was cultured from the amputation site and from the blood. An MR scan of the spine revealed a discitis at the C5/C6 level, with early destruction of the vertebral bodies but no abscess formation or spinal cord compression. A presumptive diagnosis of *Staphylococcus aureus* vertebal osteomyelitis was made and he received a six-week course of high-dose flucloxacillin and fusidic acid. Despite therapy, repeat MR scanning showed progression of the osteomyelitis involving C5 and C6 vertebral bodies, and he developed increasingly severe pain in the neck and arms. There were no features of spinal cord compression. He underwent surgical exploration and required vertebrectomies and fusion with bone from the iliac crest. Operative samples confirmed staphylococcal infection. After a further two months on high-dose antibiotics his inflammatory markers gradually settled.

A high index of suspicion is needed to make the diagnosis since back or neck pain is such a common symptom. Localised spinal tenderness can be a useful pointer, and systemic symptoms and raised inflammatory markers, including the ESR and CRP, should prompt further investigations; these should include multiple blood cultures and radiological imaging. Signs of an evolving paraparesis or quadriparesis suggest spinal cord compression, which demands urgent assessment.

Spinal MRI scanning is the investigation of choice to define the extent of the infection. Radiological evidence of involvement of the epidural space with abscess formation or confirmation of spinal compression are indications for urgent surgical exploration. In the absence of these features, treatment usually involves a prolonged course of high dose intravenous antibiotics with monitoring of clinical, radiological, and inflammatory responses. As in the case described above, this may not always be successful, and surgical debridement and arthrodesis are sometimes required.

Infection with gas-forming organisms

Patients with diabetes are at increased risk of infection from gas-forming organisms. This may affect subcutaneous tissues leading to subcutaneous gangrene, and also specific organs including the kidney and gallbladder.

Emphysematous pyelonephritis

This condition results from gas formation in the renal parenchyma as a result of severe bacterial infection of the urinary tract. A typical presentation is described in the following case report.[8]

Case Study 38

A 49-year-old woman with type 1 diabetes presented with 48 hours of rigors, vomiting, and diffuse abdominal pain. There was no past history of urinary tract disease. She was febrile and had tenderness in the lumbar region, extending to the left renal angle and iliac fossa. A clinical diagnosis of acute pyelonephritis was made and treatment with intravenous fluids, insulin, and antibiotics was started. The patient deteriorated the following day with increasing abdominal pain and tenderness to the point of left-sided abdominal rigidity. Plain abdominal X-rays showed multiple lucencies in the retroperitoneal area, and air was detected around the left kidney on ascending urography. *Escherichia coli* was cultured from blood and urine samples. Despite continued support, the patient deteriorated further, becoming confused and lethargic. She required emergency nephrectomy. The patient made a good recovery.

It is unclear why, in rare instances, these infecting organisms produce gas, although the association with poor glycaemic control has led to the suggestion that a high glucose concentration in the renal parenchyma provides an ideal substrate. *E. coli* is the commonest infecting organism, accounting for over 60% of cases. The condition should be suspected if there is no improvement after one or two days of intravenous antibiotics. Imaging of the renal tract with plain X-rays, ultrasound, or CT scanning will show gas within the renal parenchyma. Both kidneys may be involved in 10% of cases. Recommended treatment involves a prolonged course of appropriate intravenous antibiotics, together with optimal diabetic control and careful fluid balance. Nephrectomy is reserved for clinical deterioration despite medical management, but it can be life-saving.

Emphysematous cholecystitis

This is a rare complication of acute cholecystitis in which air is found in the wall and lumen of the gallbladder. In the largest reported series of over 150 cases, one-third of patients had diabetes.[9] As with acute cholecystitis, this condition presents with right upper quadrant pain, fever, and nausea although, unlike cholecystitis, it occurs more commonly in men. The diagnosis is made with plain abdominal X-rays showing gas in the gallbladder and, when it is recognised, urgent cholecystectomy is the treatment of choice, in view of the high risk of perforation. Several organisms are commonly cultured including *Clostridium perfringens* and *Escherichia coli*. Emergency cholecystectomy should be covered by antibiotics with a gram negative and anaerobic spectrum.

Skin and subcutaneous tissues

Necrotising fasciitis

This is a necrotising soft tissue infection which spreads along fascial planes, and usually results from a polymicrobial infection with anaerobic and streptococcal species of bacteria. Between 30 and 40% of cases have diabetes. It usually affects the legs, but may also affect the lower abdomen, chest, and cervical region. Presentation is usually dramatic with fever, systemic signs of toxaemia, and pain and tenderness over the affected area. Crepitation of the tissues is present in 50% of cases. The necrosis often spreads rapidly and the skin becomes increasingly discoloured with blistering. Systemic features are common including hypotension, disseminated intravascular coagulation, and organ failure.

The most important aspect of management is early recognition and appreciation of the potential severity of the condition. Surgical debridement of all necrotic tissue is the mainstay of treatment in combination with broad spectrum antibiotics. Skin grafting may be necessary once the infection has subsided. Mortality remains high at between 20 and 60%,[10] with delay in surgical intervention contributing to an increased mortality. Uncontrolled studies have suggested that hyperbaric oxygen may improve prognosis.[11]

Fournier's gangrene

This is a necrotising soft tissue infection involving the perineum and scrotum, usually presenting in a patient with signs of severe systemic illness and hypotensive shock. It is an anatomical variant of necrotising fasciitis. The following case report is typical.

Case Study 39

A 53-year-old man presented as an emergency with a two-day history of painful swelling around the groin and scrotum. He had been generally unwell, anorectic, and feverish. Two weeks previously he had been admitted for drainage of a perianal abscess, which had been completed uneventfully and was healing well. Type 2 diabetes had been diagnosed in 1994 when he was found to have moderate background retinopathy on routine eye examination. At diagnosis he was also noted to have Albustix-positive proteinuria and peripheral neuropathy. Diabetic control had been good since diagnosis with diet and metformin.

Examination revealed an indurated area over the left side of the mons pubis extending to the anal canal, and cellulitis extending to the umbilicus, into both groins and the perineum, with crepitus of the subcutaneous tissues. A diagnosis of Fournier's gangrene was made and he was taken to theatre for debridement. He required removal of necrotic subcutaneous tissue extending to the umbilicus and involving the perineal area, scrotum, and upper thighs bilaterally. Postoperatively he was managed on intensive care with high-dose antibiotics, parenteral feeding, intensive fluid replacement, and intravenous insulin by sliding scale. Cultures grew coliform organisms. His condition gradually improved and, two weeks after admission, he was accepted for split skin grafting. Final recovery of all his surgical wounds took a further three months.

As in this case, Fournier's gangrene is usually associated with perianal or urological disease, and the illness presents similar management problems to those of necrotising fasciitis. Treatment also involves urgent surgical debridement and appropriate high-dose broad spectrum antibiotics, and possibly hyperbaric oxygen if available. Skin grafting is often necessary to treat the extensive area of skin loss which often results. Even with aggressive treatment, mortality ranges between 20 and 50%.

Fungal infections

Candida vulvovaginitis

This occurs more commonly in diabetes usually as a result of poor glycaemic control with persistent glycosuria. It may be a presenting feature of newly diagnosed diabetes. Symptoms include vaginal discomfort and dyspareunia, often associated with a vaginal discharge. Treatment should include topical antifungal agents as well as trying to improve glycaemic control.

Rhinocerebral mucormycosis

This is a rare invasive infection with the *Mucor* spp. of fungus which usually occurs in immunocompromised patients. Between 50 and 70% of patients who develop rhinocerebral mucormycosis have diabetes,[12] which is usually poorly controlled. Typically the condition presents with facial oedema, proptosis, and extraocular muscle paresis. A black nasal eschar may develop with an associated bloody nasal discharge. The disease may spread to retro-orbital tissues and involve the brain. The diagnosis is made on clinical grounds and can be confirmed histologically. Treatment is difficult but should include control of diabetes, surgical removal of all involved tissues, and systemic administration of amphotericin.

Mortality is 60% when the condition complicates diabetes,[13] and survivors usually require major reconstructive surgery for facial disfigurement.

References

1 Rayfield EJ, Ault MJ, Keusch GT *et al.* Infection and diabetes, a case for glucose control. *Am J Med* 1982;72:439–50.

2 Smitherman KO, Peacock JE. Infectious emergencies in patients with diabetes mellitus. *Med Clinics N Amer* 1995;79:53–77.

3 Parfitt VJ, Hartog M Staphylococcal septicaemia in association with intracavernosal injection of alprostadil. *Diabetic Med* 1992;9:947–9.

4 Rubin J, Yu VL. Malignant otitis externa: insights into pathogenesis, clinical manifestations, diagnosis and therapy. *Am J Med* 1988;85: 391–8.

5 Lang R, Goshen S, Kitzes-Cohen R *et al.* Successful treatment of malignant external otitis with oral ciprofloxacin. *J Infect Dis* 1990;161: 537–40.

6 Jenson AG, Espersen F, Skinhoj P, Rosdahl VT, Frimodt-Moller N. Increasing frequency of vertebral osteomyelitis following staphylococcus aureus bacteraemia in Denmark 1980–1990. *J Infection* 1997;34: 113–18.

7 Baldwin N, Scott AR, Heller SR, O'Donaghue D, Tattersall RB. Vertebral and paravertebral sepsis in diabetes: an easily missed cause of backache. *Diabetic Med* 1985;2:395–7.

8 Pappas S, Pappas ThA, Sotiropoulos A, Katsadoros D. Emphysematous pyelonephritis: a case report and review of the literature. *Diabetic Med* 1993;10:574–6.

9 Mentzner RM, Golden GT, Chandler JG, Horsley JS. A comparative appraisal of emphysematous cholecystitis. *Am J Surg* 1975;129:10–15.

10 Chelsom J, Halstensen A, Hoga T *et al.* Necrotising fasciitis due to group A streptococci in western Norway: incidence and clinical features. *Lancet* 1994;344:1111–15.

11 Pizzorno R, Bonini F, Donelli A *et al.* Hyperbaric oxygen therapy in the treatment of Fournier's disease in 11 male patients. *J Urol* 1997; 158:837–40.

12 Rangel-Guerra RA, Martínez HR, Sáenz C *et al.* Rhinocerebral and systemic mucormycosis. Clinical experience with 36 cases. *J Neurolog Sci* 1996;143:19–30.

13 Blitzer A, Lawson W. Patient survival factors in paranasal sinus mucormycosis. *Laryngoscope* 1980;90:635–46.

Index